# The Best Way To Control Bladder Problems And Urinary Tract Infection Relief For Men And Women

Take back control into your life without worrying about bladder problems

# Table of Contents

# Chapter 1:
# Introduction (My Family)

I am Jeff, an engineer and a man who loves life to the fullest. Like most guys, I love sports and love the outdoors. But my passion is cooking. I am a guy who can make a meal out of scrap.

That's the reason why my high school girlfriend Margaret never hesitated to wait for me and marry me. Even though I love to cook, I never pursued my passion, but instead, I took a course that my father wanted and, of course, to land a job that could pay good money.

I graduated and was hired by one of the best firms in the city. At the age of 32, I became a junior partner in the company, and that's when Margaret and I decided to tie the knot.

I know she waited a long time for me and she has been so patient. That's why, as a wedding gift, I gave her the best wedding. I built a house for her and surprised her after the wedding. She was so happy which made me so happy as well.

Good years are beautifully spent as a married couple. We were both blessed to have two beautiful kids. Jessie, our eldest, is a pretty girl who looks exactly like me. A boy, Justin, looks like his mother.

I was earning well and was able to provide for the needs of each member of our family. That's why we were able to live harmoniously and very happily. The kids grew faster as we can imagine, and there they go, both in college already.

I am a content man married to a beautiful, wonderful, loving wife, Margaret, and two beautiful kids. I have a good-paying job that gives us a comfortable life. We live a good life, and all I can say is we are the lucky ones.

My kids are doing great in school; my eldest and only girl, Jessie, is a straight-A student and graduated at the top of her class, while my boy Justin is doing great in sports which also gave him the scholarship in college.

Cooking never left my heart; I still love cooking and cooking anything, but my specialty is Italian cuisine. My wife and I love to experiment in the kitchen. She loves to make dough because she loves to bake, pies and cakes are her things while I, on the other hand, love to make the sauces and make good pasta and calzone.

We both see to it, to have a great meal with the kids during weekends. We see that the weekend is for family time with so much fun and a home-cooked meal. Our children look forward to weekends, knowing that Margaret and I do magic in the kitchen.

Margaret and I are doing the best we can to be good parents. We both see that our children have good values and be as responsible as ever. All we wanted was that they grew as good people and help them to be the best versions of themselves.

Our eldest Jessie graduated as a civil engineer like me and is now working at one of my company's rival firms most commonly. Justin graduated with an educational degree in math major and now works in our community high school as a math teacher.

Life has been good to us, and I always dream that my kids will reach their stars and do good in their endeavors, and look at them now, they are happy with their chosen career paths.

One of a parent's greatest joys is seeing his children enjoying the perks of living a good life. Looking at my two grown and responsible kids made me more than happy. It made me feel grateful for how life has been so good.

Margaret and I are very content to see that we raise our kids well and that we have given them a chance to finish school and given them all the support they need. We are proud and happy parents.

# Chapter 2:
# My Children (Jessie and Justin)

Jessie is doing great and is becoming like me in so many ways. She is now a junior partner in her firm, young, beautiful, successful, and humble. Justin is a sagacious man, took a master's degree, graduated, and is now taking his PhD.

I know that Jessie has been dating guys, and my boy Justin had a few girlfriends. But now, they both are very much in love with two great creatures that Margaret and I adore, Tanner and Patricia.

Even though they have their places now, they never forget to spend the weekend with us. No matter how busy they are, they ensure that the weekend is reserved to bond with the family.

They spend the night with us, and I like it because it is a chance that the four of us get to bond. I am the king of the kitchen, and I love cooking for my family in those times. Be their dad again, and be the head of the family again.

As I was planning the menu for next weekend, I got a call from Jessie. She said she would be bringing three companies, including Tanner's best friend. As I dropped the phone, it rang again, and it was Justin, this time saying the same thing.

They both will bring their partners plus guests. Oh well, I said the more, the merrier; they are practically family.  My menu will have to be for more people, not just the four of us.

The weekend arrives, Margaret and I are too busy preparing. She is baking her famous apple pie and making her favorite potato salad, and I was making the best tuna pesto, calzone, and my famous ratatouille.

It took us hours to prepare the best dish for our kids, and we know that their company will love it too. They arrive in time for lunch with their partners, and to my surprise, both Tanner and Patricia's parents are there.

The meal was excellent, sharing it with my loved ones and their loved ones as well. As Margaret serves coffee, Justin says that Patricia has a beautiful surprise. Jessie was shouting that she had a surprise too, "I must say first as I am the eldest", she said. That's what I love about my kids, they always love to surprise us.

Margaret was serving coffee now, well actually she is famous for her coffee, she made the best cappuccino. Both parents of Tanner and Patricia looked forward to it and, of course, her favorite apple pie. Tanner and Jessie stood up and were excited, saying, "Mom, Dad, we are planning to get married." That is why Tanner's parents are here because he proposed to my daughter last Monday. They are planning to get married in June.

She was telling us how Tanner proposed. It was somewhat romantic. She said that Tanner called her to meet him at the dentist because he was afraid to undergo his root canal appointment. His tooth was bugging him for the week, and even Jessie can't sleep because of him whining.

She never thought that Tanner and the dentist were only setting her up. She hurriedly went to the dentist that afternoon, and when she arrived, he was already in the seat and was being treated. The dentist told Jessie a slight problem because he found something unusual in his gums. He urges Jessie to look at it.

Knowing my daughter is inquisitive about everything, she immediately looks at it. As she was taking a peak, she immediately asked the dentist, "what is that?". She saw a shining thing at Tanners in between teeth.

The dentist handed the mirror and one of the tools, and as she was looking at it, she shouted, "Oh My God" She saw a diamond ring. Then as she was still screaming, Tanner knelt into his knees, asking her, "Jessie, I love you, will you be my wife?".

She was telling it with so much enthusiasm that all of us were giggling. In my daughter's eyes, I can see that she is delighted and that I only want what is best for her. Tanner is a great guy, and I know that he loves my daughter so much deep in my heart.

Margaret was tearing up, and I could see that the love of my life was thrilled too. She raised our children well. It's all because they both grew up with good values and were very loving.

The day has come, and my little girl is all grown up and getting married. I never thought that this day would come so fast. It seems like yesterday when I held her in my hand and fed her.

Margaret was so excited by saying that she would be the one to help Jessie with the wedding details. My wife is great with the little details. She always sees to it that everything is in order.

As we are busy giving all our suggestions about the upcoming wedding in 3 months, my youngest then blurts out, "What about me? Don't you want to hear what I am about to say?".

We all laugh, and Margaret, just as the best mother, is asked, "What is it, honey?"

He then said, "I know that you are pleased and all, no offense, sister, but we have the best news for all of you too." He then smiled very timidly and said, "Mom, Dad, Sis, Patricia, and I are going to have a baby." A sudden silence was on the table and then suddenly Margaret shouted excitedly and said: "I'm going to be a grandma?!"

From that moment, Margaret was very joyful, and I, on the other hand, still couldn't believe what had just happened. Indeed, it was great news; I cannot express how I feel, knowing that my kids are both happy and very much in love with their partners. And that I am going to be a grandad gives me the most overwhelming feeling.

As we parents, we're talking about the details of the wedding. Suddenly, Justin came out, and He and Tanner had a great idea. He called Jessie and Patricia, spoke to them, and then came to us. It was hilarious. They both agreed to have a double wedding. I can't believe what I am hearing, but it was the best decision ever.

Both my kids think alike, and since they were young, they share the same familiar things and enjoy each other's company. Margaret and I don't have a problem with both of them. We did our best to raise our children well, but I give all the credits to my loving wife.

Looking back when they reach their teen years, they always take care of each other. They helped their mom with all chores in the house constantly. Make sure that it is all done at the end of the day.

Jessie, being the eldest, is a responsible girl, and she always looks after Justin, who is only less than two years younger than her. I don't know how Margaret raised them, but I like that they don't keep secrets from each other.

Margaret and I never experienced that our children were in trouble. Jessie is a consistent straight-A student like her mother. She excels in many ways, like art club and drama club, while my boy is trendy for being handsome and a math whiz. Both of them are very smart and very reliable.

They graduated from high school with flying colors. Having these two beautiful kids is a dream for Margaret and me. They all have their flaws, but it is very tolerable and prevalent for me.

Like Jessie, a significant mess in the kitchen when preparing some food, but it is spotless in the bathroom. On the other hand, Justin is immaculate in the kitchen and loves to do the dishes while leaving the bathroom like a hurricane passes by.

They both can be hard-headed sometimes, but gladly they are afraid of their mom. Margaret may have the softest voice in the world, but when she says it's enough, it means it is enough.

You can be grounded in a week if she says so. And I am telling you when she says you cannot go out, and you cannot. She will guard you like a hawk. I am more like the coolest dad in the world. I hang out with my kids like I am one of them. Justin's friends love to hang out and jam with me and my guitar and love my pizza during weekends.

Although one incident with Justin scares the hell out of me, my boy fell in love when he was a freshman in college. He was so lost when the girl turned her down.

He went home and said that he didn't want to go back to school anymore because the girl was in his class, and he was devastated that she didn't like her.

Justin was depressed for a week or two. He just stays in his room

6

and lies in bed for days. I don't want to go out and don't want to talk to anybody.

At first, I thought it was only regular for boys to be dumped by girls. Of course, I haven't experienced it because the first girl I fell in love with married me. But as days pass by, it seems alarming because he doesn't want to eat and doesn't want to bathe. He stares at the ceiling. I told Margaret that we should bring him to a psychiatrist or whatever, but my loving wife just calmly said, "Leave it to me."

All he needs is his mother to be back on his feet again. They had just spent an overnight camping trip in the lake, and the next day he was smiling again. And after three days, he went back to school again.

It is like she works miracles for all of us. And then She only reminds me to talk to our son once in a while and be mindful of whatever issue He has been dealing with, and She can do magic.

After that, Justin seemed to be all right, and the following year, he met Patricia, and the rest is history for both of them. He continued his studies until he graduated with flying colors too. I am so proud of my son. He is a good son and a good person too. Now, he is a good husband and a good father as well.

My children are the best. They both grow up with a fabulous mother and, of course, a supporting dad. I know that they will live the life that Margaret and I dreamed of; I can affirm that.

They are both lucky to have their partners by their side. My kids are great parents too. We raised good people with good values, loving, affectionate, and strong warriors like their mother.

# Chapter 3:
# The Double Wedding

Jessie is the best sister to Justin. That is why it didn't surprise me when she agreed to share her wedding with her brother.

Justin has been worrying about what Patricia might feel unimportant if the wedding is held after birth. So, knowing well that his sister can't say "no" to him, he asked us to gather for a family meeting and talk about the possibility of having two weddings in one day.

Margaret instantly agreed to Justin's proposed plan as the loving and supportive mother she always is. It has always been her dream to organize our children's weddings. So, not only will this fulfil her life-long dream, but it will also be one unique celebration not many families get to have and enjoy.

Jessie looked worried at first; she was concerned about how Patricia would react to his brother's double wedding plan. So, before saying "yes" she asked Justin to talk to Patricia first, and she would go talk to Tanner.

After successfully discussing the plan with their partners, they were finally happy to inform their mom and me that the double wedding was a go! They were so excited about how they got to share the happiest day of their lives.

However, beneath all the daydreaming and excitement, reality struck us hard when we realized that we only have more or less two months left to prepare for their weddings because we want to have it before Patricia's 1st trimester ends.

Justin started panicking all over the place. On the other hand, Jessie and Tanner were so hands-on with the wedding preparations, they even insisted on paying for everything. I was so proud of my little girl, but Margaret and I decided to pitch in for the wedding, so we told the kids that we would be the ones making their wedding cakes.

A month has passed, only a few more weeks left before the wedding. Everyone was starting to feel mixed emotions, especially the couples who were both excited and anxious about their marriage. But luckily for all of us, Margaret was there to keep everyone calm.

She was the one who made sure that we followed the pre-wedding events schedule and still had enough time to look good during the parties. Having a double wedding that involves both your kids can be a handful. It was very tiring having to cook for different groups of friends of each couple, but I managed it by having Margaret by my side.

There was only a week left before the wedding, and I didn't expect the nervousness I felt a few weeks ago to intensify. I had this sudden urge to pee all the time, but I didn't mind because I knew it was only nerves and excitement from all the fiasco around me.

Also, I don't have the time to worry about myself because I have to make sure that my wife, kids, and soon-to-be kids are in good hands. We decided to check in the hotel three days before the wedding to settle in and prepare for the wedding of the decade.

Families from both sides have flown in to attend the wedding. The brides have scheduled their spa day with their best friends, and the grooms went last-minute shopping for shoes and belts with their buddies.

Everyone was busy and elated at the same time. You could hear laughter and chatters echoing in the hotel lobby as the couple friends and our families gathered to have small conversations to catch up with each other.

Then, here comes the day everyone was waiting for, Justin and Jessie's double wedding day. I cannot describe how I felt that day. I was so emotional and happy to be able to experience the happiest day in the lives of my two precious gems.

Margaret was happy too, and even when she was crying every 5 minutes, I could feel it in my heart that she was ecstatic. Despite all the emotions felt at that time, we could still compose ourselves and managed to make two 3-layered wedding cakes for both our children.

The wedding was a blast! Both our kids are now officially married, and all I wish for them is that they get to spend all their days with the one they truly love because that's what Margaret and I have been doing all these years.

The reception party was somehow wild, but of course, Patricia has to be careful because she is pregnant, so we decided to accompany her back to the room together with Justin. We are allowing them to have their alone time so that they can rest after a whole day of stress, happiness, and celebration of love.

On the other hand, Jessie and Tanner are having the best party moment in their life as a married couple. They were dancing all over the reception with their best buddies beside them.

The guests were enjoying the party as well. They repeatedly praised Margaret and me for putting together a successful double wedding, cooking good food, and baking the wedding cakes.

I was grinning the whole time, I glanced at my beautiful wife, and I went to ask her to slow dance with me. It felt like the day of our wedding too. After these years, I realized how I'm still madly in love with Margaret. We danced the night away and ended it by sending our 2nd lovebirds to their love nest.

It was comforting to see and feel that all went well the next day. We had our first family brunch at the hotel restaurant, and it was nice seeing my kids so happy together with their partners. Justin and Patricia also gave us some great news, the lab results are in, and they are having twins. They have been suspecting for a while now, but they wanted to be sure before telling us the news.

It was a happy day for all of us until I noticed how Margaret kept on going back and forth to the bathroom. I went after her and tried asking her what was wrong, but she just smiled and told me that all the food she was eating must be taking its toll on her because she felt like she was having heartburn.

I smiled back to reassure her and told her to tell me if it bothered her. Then, we went back to the dining table and continued the fun conversations with our children. We were having a good time when I suddenly felt a pinch of pain in the lower portion of my stomach. I excused myself and went to the restroom.

I left the table for about 5 minutes until Jessie went after me, telling me that Margaret had fainted. We rushed back to our table, and we saw that the hotel personnel were already giving Margaret first aid.

After a few seconds, she finally regained consciousness. Jessie and Justin insisted that we should still take her to the hospital, but Margaret insisted that she was just tired and all she wanted to do was go back to our room and rest.

Assuring our kids that I would take care of their mother, I took Margaret back to our room and prepared the bed for her to rest for the night. As I assisted her, I noticed how weak she was. I was apprehensive, so I waited for her to fall asleep, then I called the kids for an emergency family meeting about their mom.

Jessie blamed herself for asking too much help from Margaret and causing her to suffer from overfatigue, but Justin and I were just quiet until she asked us what we were thinking at that moment.

"Mom's been acting weird lately, and she keeps on holding her chest as if it is hurting her." Justin shared. Then, he looked at me, telling me that his observation started long before the double wedding preparations began.

Jessie looked at me with worry in her eyes. "Dad? Do you think Mom is sick and she's keeping it from us?" she asked. I reached out for her hand and held it tightly. I didn't know what to say to the children because I didn't know what was happening.

We went silent for a while, and then I sighed. "Let's not worry right away. Maybe your Mom was just tired after the big event yesterday," I told them. Then, I sent them back to their respective rooms to rest after a long day.

Justin and Jessie's voices echoed into my ears as I walked back to our room. That's when it occurred to me, what is happening to my wife? Is she sick? Is she keeping it to herself? Is she even aware of the things that are happening to her?

Then, I remembered how Margaret told me minutes before she fainted that she thought she was suffering from heartburn. I was worried for my wife, but we had to be sure first. That's when I knew that we had to take a trip to the hospital and have her checked.

# Chapter 4:
# My Grandchildren

Today marks the 6th month anniversary of my children's wedding. We were all excitedly waiting for the twins to come out to the world finally. Margaret and I kept ourselves busy by going crazy on buying every baby stuff we could ever find.

Jessie and Tanner were excited to meet their nieces or nephews too. We still don't know the gender yet because Justin and Patricia wanted it to surprise us. So, we patiently waited for the new addition to the family.

Margaret was back on her feet too. After that incident the day after the wedding, we decided to extend our stay at the hotel to give her a few more days to regain her strength, and she did.

After our three-day extended vacation, we went home, and everything returned to normal. Now, we are happily waiting for the call from Justin telling us that we are officially grandparents.

After the wedding, the kids moved out of the house, and since then, it's just Margaret and me spending our days baking and gardening together. It was fun because it took us back to the days when it was just the two of us in the big house without children with messy hands running around.

But we missed those days, so we are patiently looking forward to experiencing those days again by the time the twins are big enough to run and get messy. Oh, how much fun would that be, being able to hear babies giggling and crying in the house again? After so many years that Margaret and I were used to hearing my two children, Jessie and Justin, squabbling and arguing with each other about the remote control.

It was five o'clock in the morning when Margaret and I got awoken by the sound of our telephone. We got up, and she answered it. It was Jessie, and she called to say that she and Tanner were coming to pick us up. "Justin called earlier. The twins are coming!" she shrieked.

We immediately put on our coats, and while waiting for Jessie and Tanner, I noticed that I had an unread message on my phone. Justin said that he had taken Patricia to the hospital because she was already experiencing contractions. I showed it to Margaret, who was busy checking if we had brought the right clothes for the twins.

I can say that my wife and I are more than just excited for the coming of our grandchildren. We were ready to enter this new stage of our lives. I grabbed the identical bears we bought for the twins and then waited for Jessie and Tanner outside the house.

After the car arrived, we jumped right in and proceeded to go to the hospital. We saw Justin right away, and he told us that Patricia is still in the delivery room and that the doctors haven't given him any updates yet.

I can see how my son is worried for his wife and kids, but as much as I want to comfort him, I can't because my bladder is bothering me. I have this tingling feeling and have to excuse myself to go to the restroom.

Margaret saw the discomfort on my face and asked if I wanted her to accompany me to the restroom. Still, I assured her that I was okay, and it was probably just nerves because of mixed emotions of too much excitement and worry for my daughter-in-law and grandchildren.

I went to the restroom, and the tingling sensation that I was feeling turned into this excruciating pain just below the abdomen. I was curling up on the restroom floor to try and position myself comfortably to ease the pain.

Then, the pain went away, and I was able to wash my face with some water and decided to go back to the waiting area to comfort my family. As soon as I went back, the doctor was already talking to Justin, and from afar, I could see that it was great news.

My son is a father! I can't believe it, I used to hold him in my arms, and now, I am watching him juggling two babies in his arms. One girl and one boy were added as new members of our family.

As I gazed at everyone glancing at Ari and Adam, I smiled. It was a great day for the family, and I hope that happy days like this will continue. And to dismay, this might be the last happy moment that my family will experience in a while because the following days will be challenging for us, for me primarily.

# Chapter 5:
# Margaret (Till Death do us Part)

That moment that I laid my eyes on her was the most unforgettable moment for me. She is lovely in so many ways. Her smile is like an energy that can pull you on your seat. The sound of her voice is very light as the air that whistles on your ear. Her soft tone makes you wonder if she knows how to shout.

Her red hair is like the leaves you can see in autumn; her light complexion is like the sun in your eyes. She is perfect to me. I cannot imagine she will be my wife.

Margaret is the type of person that always speaks herself. She is very vocal about her emotions and never ashamed to express her feelings towards any incident or anybody. My parents adore her that every time we misunderstand, my mother always makes a way to patch things up again.

She is a good cook and always finds time to bake for my parents and me. As my mother used to say, she is a good catch and a whole package.

She was there in my life the whole time when I was in high school, college, my struggles, my pain when my mom and dad died in a car crash, and all the happy moments in my life.

Margaret was present. I never regretted a single day in my life because she was there. I love her with all my heart and my soul. I cannot imagine my life without her.

I married her when I was stable, both in my job and financially. I gave her the best wedding ever, I built a house for her, and she made it home.

She was so organized and ensured that she never forgot anything, especially with me. I can still remember that my alarm clock is the aroma of her brewed coffee and the smell of my breakfast. I remember it all too well.

She gave me two beautiful children, and she was the strongest, loving mother I have ever known. She makes sure that the kids are well taken care of and never forgets to do her obligation as a wife to me. She makes sure that the excitement and spark are always there.

She makes sure we communicate both in words and in mind. I am proud to say that I never cheated on her and, it never crossed my mind to be attracted to other women.

The only flaw of Margaret is that she never talked about any physical pain or if she is not feeling well. She hides if she is sick or never shows us if she is feeling any pain. She doesn't want anybody to be worried about her. She doesn't want me to worry.

That's what I hate about her—never been so vocal about her feelings towards sickness. She is one hard-headed woman who thinks she knows it all and hides her feelings about it when it comes to illness. That's why even her parents and sisters hate her for being like that.

The first time I notice something odd about her is when she makes excuses at the children's wedding. As I watched her put on her gown, I asked her, "Why are you losing weight? I don't like you that thin, and you look a little pale".

As great as she is, she uses her soft voice saying, I am just being silly. She started to throw up a couple of times and started to feel dizzy most of the time. Her weight is decreasing, and I can see that She is in the best shape most of the time.

She keeps on saying that the wedding preparation is one of the reasons why She is losing weight. The stress, the excitement, and the waiting are always some of the reasons. She gives. Margaret is a person who is very keen on details, a perfectionist, and a hands-on kind of person.

After the wedding, Margaret became a little bit slow. She sometimes forgot everything, even her usual daily routine. She is paler and not eating that much. I was so worried that I insisted we should see a doctor. The minute the doctor saw her, all blood samples were taken, and the doctor requested an MRI.

The results came, and we were referred to an Oncologist. I will never forget that day; I think my heart stopped for a second when the oncologist said that she had stage two breast cancer. We were given choices, chemo, or other treatments.

It dramatically impacts us, especially our children, because they are very close with their mother. Margaret never mentioned anything or showed any symptoms. But I know her too well, and I know she is hiding it from us. She never wants us to worry, and she looks strong so that we won't think that she is suffering that much.

It is like Margaret wants us to see that she is indestructible. She is always calm and has an answer to everything. Our children grew up very well taken care of, especially if they are sick. Margaret is very keen, visits the pediatrician, has round-the-clock medication, is well prepared for a healthy meals and doesn't sleep, being beside them all the time.

They grew up strong, aware, and conscious of what they eat because their mother always reminds them of the Dos and the Don'ts. She is the best mother for them and the best person for me. Now I don't know what to do and how to take care of her knowing she is very sick.

I keep blaming myself for not giving her all the attention she needs. I am a busy man running a company. Being a good dad and a good provider, I doubt I am a good husband. I felt like I had neglected the person whom I loved the most. Now I am denying that she will be gone in a blink of an eye.

To get the best results, the doctor immediately started the treatments. Chemo is a little harsh with Margaret, and She has all the side effects. Vomiting became worse every day, and she could not get out of bed most of the days. She is exhausted most of the time and doesn't want to be touched. She lies in bed and sleeps most of the day. That is so not Margaret.

Months and days passed by, and she became sicker and sicker. As if the chemo is not working. The good thing about Margaret is that she is trying really hard to eat and stand even though she is too weak. She shows us that she can do it even though she can't. She has the will to live.

The moment of truth came as the doctors were about to see if the chemo affected her. She is set to get tested again. Then, there it is, bad results. Her body is not responding to the treatments. I am out of words listening to the doctor. It is like someone stabbing me in the heart, and the pain is unbearable.

The doctors were suggesting another way of treatment, but Margaret said no. That was the worst. I was mortified that I kept on arguing with her and became hysterical. All I could hear was my voice shouting and pleading with her to reconsider. But to my dismay, she just kept on saying no.

We went home with a silent treatment with each other. I was not too fond of the fact that Margaret was giving up. I married a strong-willed woman and a very hard-headed one too.

She is so stubborn and always believes in what is on her mind. I know that she grew up being independent and all but this time, I want to decide what is best for her and make sure that she receives all the best treatment and medication.

I talked to the kids to convince their mother to give it another try. I was hoping they could change her mind and make her seek a second opinion and do what the doctors suggested, but again, she said no. Jessie insists and begs her mom, just telling her to give it another try, but Margaret shakes her head, saying no.

As we were having dinner, Margaret gave her reason why she wouldn't try other treatments. She said that it is a waste of money, time, effort and that she would like to be remembered as an active woman and not a sickly one. She would want to spend it with us and not at the hospital.

I feel like someone is punching my chest. Margaret knows that our retirement money is gone and that she doesn't want me to worry about financial matters. I will do everything for her, and now she is giving it up. She just grabbed my hand and said, "It will be okay!".

After that moment, Justin had his PhD. and was offered the job, and Jessie got her new promotion and got pregnant. The twins are growing fast, and I think it helped Margaret because she was happy that day. It brings her stamina, and she looks forward to waking up every day.

Justin and Patricia came back to the house after returning from the hospital. It made Margaret happier. I can see her smiling more often now. She became unstoppable, going back and forth to give Patricia a hand with the twins.

It became clearer to me now why she didn't want to spend more of her time at the hospital. She is cooking again for us and taking good care of our grandchildren.

Months passed, and the horrific day came. It was a Saturday morning, and I decided to cook for us. Jessie and Tanner are spending the weekend with us. So, it is time to make the most incredible pizza and calzone for today.

I was about to kiss my lovely wife when she grabbed and hugged me, saying, "I love you, thank you for making me happy!" She gave me the sweetest smile and wink. I just kissed her passionately.

While Justin and I were preparing in the kitchen, Jessie and Tanner arrived, and she brought a new comfortable pillow for her mom. She hurriedly went upstairs, and all we could hear was her scream. Margaret was not breathing, we hastily brought her to the hospital, and she was declared dead on arrival.

That was it, there she goes!

She was saying goodbye to me that morning. The children were devastated. They kept on saying that they weren't able to say goodbye. When Jessie saw her mother, Margaret told her that she would be okay and loved her so much.

Justin was when Margaret said to him, "You are becoming the best man like your dad; keep it up. I will always be here for you because I love you. " It is all a sign that She is saying goodbye.

The love of my life is gone. Till death do us part. We will lay her to rest, and it is the saddest day for my children and me. All I can think about now is how my life would be without her? At the funeral, all our family and friends were present.

The moment was when Margaret's sisters were telling us about how good she was, was so sad. All the good memories of Margaret were mentioned by those who remember her, A beautiful person inside and out. She is indeed correct. She will be remembered as a good, happy, light of the party person, not a sick, hopeless one.

# Chapter 6:
# Coping and Picking Up the Pieces

Margaret died a slow death. She spent the rest of her days with all of us and didn't suffer that much, and until she closed her eyes, she was still the same woman I fell in love with over the years.

From the day she was diagnosed, Margaret never showed any sign of pain. For the past years that she has been suffering, she still never stopped doing what she loves.

We still celebrate the family day every weekend, and the kids always see to it that we never fail to bond. The grandchildren spend extra time with grandmother, especially if Margaret wants to cook or bake cakes for them.

She never shows them that she is experiencing pain. She once told me that," I want my grandchildren to remember me as the coolest, happy, and strong, not sick."

I know that is not the same Margaret; she lost her long beautiful hair from chemotherapy, yet she still tries to look good for us. Her weight drops down if I hold her by the waist. It is like a fragile thing that I am afraid I might break.

Despite that, her appearance and stamina are not the same. Still, she is the happy pill that I married.

I went home to an empty house each day. I feel like my world is crumbling down. I can feel her presence, but I can't see her, driving me crazy. I eat alone now, and most of the time, I just don't eat at all.

I know that I am letting myself go, and worse, I have been drinking a lot lately. I want to go home very tired and tipsy so that all I can do is sleep. In that way, I feel less pain.

My children are worried and my friends as well. They notice that I am not myself anymore. My job is at stake, too, because I am not performing well at the office.

I have turned down so many projects because I feel like I can't do it.

My self-confidence drops down, and I am beginning to doubt myself. I feel useless and very lonely at the same time.

Jessie is about to have her second child, so she hasn't visited for two weeks now. Justin, Patricia, and the twins spend summertime with their parents in the countryside, and they haven't come back, so I am all alone.

The drinking and smoking problem is starting, and it is the only thing that makes me company most of the time. I never imagined my life without Margaret, I never felt so alone, and it broke my heart.

My boss and mentor called me up in his office the next day. He is like a second father to me. He believes in me and has never doubted me since the first day he hired me.

He said to me, "What are you doing with your life? Do you think Margaret would love seeing you like this?" For the first time since Margaret died, I burst into tears. I have been holding my tears because I want her to see I am strong and don't want her to know that I am losing my mind.

My boss gave me a vacation to figure things out. He said I needed some time to heal. He had given me the advice to deal with Margaret's death because he never saw me moving on. I took his advice and took time off from work. I spent time with my friends and went fishing and drinking with them.

One of my friends suggested that to cope with the loneliness over Margaret's death, and I should travel or do something I love. He said that Margaret would love me to do it. And then It hit me, and I can't live like this! I have to find a way to cope and prove to Margaret that I am the strong man she marries.

I thought about my decision for quite some time, and I am sure I will do. The following weeks were crucial because I didn't know if my boss would be happy about it, but I had already made up my mind. I haven't talked to my children, so I don't know their reaction either.

The minute I arrived at the office; I knew that this day would change my life forever. As soon as my boss arrived, I hurriedly went to his office. At first, I didn't know where to start, but there was no turning back because I had already made up my mind. "I will quit my job!"

As I handed my resignation letter, I explained to my boss that life is not easy for me lately. If I don't do something about it, I will go crazy. I told him that I ran it through my mind repeatedly to make sure that I was making the right decision.

To my amazement, his reaction is the other way around from what I thought. He said he would never doubt my plans because he knows me too well. I will excel in whatever endeavor I choose.

And before I could say the last words, he just put his hands on my shoulders and said, "Feel free to come back if you want to work with us again."

I went home knowing that I made the most significant decision ever, but I am hopeful that Margaret will be proud if I succeed in these new plans.

I have to pick up the pieces in my life, or I will linger in my loneliness and be nothing more than a worthless person to my children and grandchildren. That night, I called my kids and asked them to come because we had to sit down and discuss important matters.

That night I wasn't able to sleep. All I did was wander around the house, and every corner had Margaret's memories. I can still smell her, and I can still hear her voice. She laughs, and I can feel her.

I built that house for her, but she polished it, decorated it, and made it a home for our children and me. She is the light of that big house, and now that light is gone. The inside of the house looks dark, and all the areas feel empty and lifeless.

The following day, both my children will come. It was the first time we saw each other after Margaret's funeral, and it's been two months. When the car arrived, I was like a child running towards the door to see who came first.

It was Justin, Patricia, and the Twins. Then, Tanner's car came too. Boy, my only daughter, Jessie, is so beautiful in her term month. Harley is growing into a pretty girl. I was so happy to see my children and grandchildren again. It seems like forever.

As we were having lunch, I was so quiet that Jessie was staring at me, saying, "Dad are you okay?" I have many things going on in my mind. I don't know where to start; Margaret usually has the first say regarding decision-making, but now I am left alone.

I cry a lot now. Even, looking at her empty seat seems to break my heart, but I have to be a man and let my children know my plans.

I told my children that I decided that can change our lives forever. They were so eager to listen to me when I told them that I had left my job and planned to put up a restaurant in the city.

I also told them I was planning to sell the house and had already found an agent to deal with the house. I am trying to explain to them my dilemma and that I cannot live here anymore. I want to move on, and this is the only way I know to forget all that had happened.

They were all speechless, and they didn't know that I was going through so much. My children never argued about my decision. Although Justin thinks I have to think about the house, he knows that I am doing the right thing for whatever it's worth.

I told them that the restaurant is their mother's dream and that she would be happy If this pushed it through. She has always been supportive of my dream to invest in a family business. It was actually our dream together. She will be the one in charge of the baking and management, then I'll be in charge of the main dishes and inventory.

As we were about to finish discussing my plans, Jessie's bag of water broke.

Tanner and I rush her to the hospital, and after an hour, I am a granddad of a charming baby girl who looks exactly like her grandma, and Jessie named her Margaret.

When I first held her in my hand, I could see that Margaret was looking at me through her eyes. From that moment on, I knew I could do things right. I know that she will be proud of me and be with me throughout my new journey.

A week after, someone bought the house, and I found an apartment near the city. Leaving it all behind was the hardest thing to do, but I had to go on. All the memories in that house are both delighted and sad.

I can't live with it anymore, and I have to leave it to continue living a life with new hope and perspective. The beginning is always the hardest. But with the support of my children and good friends, it seems that all is well.

I bought a place near the beach for the restaurant. It was a lovely spot because it overlooks the sea and the refreshing breeze. It is very accessible and only within walking distance to the park and the library.

I know that if it's meant to be, all will fall into its place. No matter how hard it was, everything was in order within six months. I was about to open the restaurant and take a test drive from all the machines and the oven.

Having my family and friends around seems to be the best part because it all flows perfectly. Jessie takes time to interview the staff, Justin and my friends take charge of all the kitchen stuff and utensils to be used, Tanner helps with the renovation, Patricia helps with all the paperwork.

I am just one who bosses around and looks at all the details in the restaurant that must be arranged. I designed the whole restaurant with Margaret's taste, of course. Working hand in hand is making things done in a minimal period. It was the best therapy for all of us.

The name of the restaurant is "Maggie's Ristorante Italiano." I want it to sound like Margaret's personality, relaxed, happy, homey, motherly. It offers the best Italian pizzas, calzone, six varieties of pasta, and my famous ratatouille.

We also offer all kinds of coffee, beer, freshly squeezed fruit juices, and some desserts. The restaurant's ambiance is very soothing, amicable, and cozy. There is an excellent view of the sea and the air, so crisp you can feel the love.

Being busy for the past months stopped my drinking and smoking problems. It also helps with my loneliness and my anxiety. I am coping well, and I know that I made the right decision to push through these plans.

My new apartment also helps because I go home with no memories of Margaret, all I do is sleep there, and that's it. It seems like all the beginning to be well for me. It is not that I am over it, but I am getting there.

The day is almost here. I am so excited because I really put a lot of effort into this restaurant. The whole family is all coming together and two days from now, we will finally start the business properly. Jessie made arrangements for the first day to be a blast.

On opening night, great exciting events like free concerts from local bands, free drinks, and more freebies like coffee mugs and cups. I am very excited and overwhelmed at the same time because all our hard work paid off. The time has come. It is the moment I've been waiting for a long time! I know Margaret will be proud of us and our efforts. .

The opening day was a success. Many came and enjoyed the food and the place as well. It was a blast, and we earned more than we expected. All the family members are there and Family of both sides of my children's partners.

My children and I were touched seeing Margaret's family being there too. I am so happy with the outcome that I knew in my heart that moving on was the best thing I did.

Being busy for the past month helped me with my drinking and smoking problems. Being tired at the end of the day doesn't give me time to cry over Margaret's death. Being excited about the outcome gives me a reason to get up each day and gives me much hope in my heart.

Coping with Margaret's death is not easy. Moving on is hard. Picking up the pieces is like dying and living again. I love my wife so much that there is no point in living a life without her.

I became useless after she died. I almost forgot that I still have my children and grandchildren to look into the future. I still have a beautiful life because of the people left behind who love me and look up to me.

I have friends who continually get my back no matter what life brings me. I never realized all of this until I felt so useless during that time. I have been a very positive person ever since, but after Margaret's death, I became so negative that I couldn't even work without thinking I would fail.

The Idea of building this restaurant helps me see the light after darkness. I am eager to help myself cope, move on, and pick up the pieces. Selling the house is also a great idea because I will not linger in Margaret's memory in all the house corners. Her scent that is still in our room makes me suffer, and all the things that she left behind make me sick to my stomach.

Now, I have other things to think about from now on. The restaurant, the customers, the next day's menu, and what else I should do to make it more appealing to people. My children never left my side, and they are giving their time even now. I have many things to be thankful for each day.

I am beginning to rise again. I am beginning to see the light again. I use Margaret's memory as a stepping stone to living life again. Pursuing our restaurant's dream gives me the courage to dream again. Her memory is the only weapon I use to stand up to my feet again.

She is my inspiration, she is my strength, and Margaret is why I am doing what I am doing right now. Even though she is not around anymore, I know she watched me live our dream.

This dream is for her, for our children and grandchildren. I want to build this because I want them to remember Margaret even when I am gone.

I know that I made the right decision about quitting my job and putting up this restaurant. I know someone up there guided me to do this. Not only did it help me to move on, but I found myself again.

The Restaurant was my redemption, and Margaret is my inspiration. The passion and love for cooking are in my heart. No matter how successful I am in my chosen career, it is in my blood, and I cannot let go of it.

So now I promise Margaret that I will be the strong man she married again.

I will go on with my life again and be inspired by her memory. I will take care of our offspring and their offspring like she did when she was still alive.

I promise that I will do my best to build a legacy we once dreamed of when Margaret was still alive. I will do my best to live the life she wants me to live, and I will live once again even though she is not there anymore. I will live for her and my children.

# Chapter 7:
# Here Comes My Bladder

I know those bladder problems are most common in women. And it doesn't mean that being a man is an excuse to get this kind of problem. I know that I haven't been good to my health when Margaret got sick, and by the time she died, I became harsh to myself.

I started to drink and smoke almost every day. I ate unhealthy food like junk foods and take outs and didn't exercise during that time. Although I had symptoms by the time Margaret was sick, I kept ignoring it, adding the stress it had given me and the worries centered on Margaret alone.

There are times that it is painful to pee, and it keeps on bugging me, especially during the night-time, but it sometimes goes away, so I didn't mind it at all. I know that the feeling is not normal anymore, but I don't give any importance to it. I know I have a history of UTI, and I was diagnosed, but paying too much attention to myself is the last thing on my mind.

The doctor prescribed some medicine and advised me to take it diligently in order to be cured, but I always forgot about it. I have so many things going on in my mind than thinking about myself.

I hadn't felt it for almost four years until the restaurant peaked and when Mari came into my life. I already felt something before we went out on a date, and I ignored it again until the day when we were supposed to spend our time together for the first time, and it bugged me that my bladder was making a scene.

Although it ruined our first kiss, it is an attention seeker. I am just lucky that Mari was so excellent that day. She asked me what was wrong and very eager to know what was going on. I feel so comfortable telling her and talking about that stuff to her. I am glad that she understood my situation because she experienced it herself.

I told her that the first time I experienced it was when Margaret was undergoing chemo. I almost forgot to take care of myself during that time. All I think was Margaret's sake. She has my full attention during that time. All I wanted was for her to be okay and to feel better.

The signs that I felt that time was:

1) Tingling sensation whenever I urinate.
2) The color of my urine is darker.
3) Frequent urination, especially at night.
4) Fever.
5) Chills during sleep
6) Blood in my urine

These are the first few signs, and the feeling of discomfort is there all the time. I never realized that it was getting alarming. The moment that I was having pain was when I sought medical help. I was cured, and the doctor gave me antibiotics.

And now, I am having the same signs and symptoms again. Ignoring what I felt before is okay, but now I have a new chance with love, and I don't want to ruin the latest chapters of my life with Mari just because of my bladder. I am thankful to Mari because she is a big help, and she convinces me to see a doctor again.

And I made the right decision now seeing a urologist, and I was glad. I keep on asking him why it keeps on coming back. I told the doctor that I first experienced it when Margaret was sick and having chemotherapy. Due to a lack of self-attention, I began to feel the signs and symptoms that I ignored.

I don't have any idea that there is such a thing as recurrence and that there is a possibility that men can also acquire it. I have neglected that I am not getting any younger and taking care of myself.

Now I am aware, and I am well informed about bladder problems. And what to do and not to do. And how to prevent it. To eat forbidden foods and to exercise regularly. My friend introduced a product that I can buy online and, in the store, online.

The name of the product is Flotrol natural bladder support. I have been taking Flotrol for my overactive bladder. Since my recurrence, I have been using it, and I have better bladder control. With all the natural ingredients, there are no side effects, and you can buy it without a prescription.

It is awe-inspiring because it is very effective. My friend and His wife have been using it for more than a year, and they can attest that it is effective and impressive.

They have been suffering from bladder problems ever since and have a recurrence. Still, after taking Flotrol and following the proper intake, they no longer have the urgency to go to the bathroom, especially at night.

I, myself, can affirm that. After taking it for three days, I can feel the effects. I no longer wake up at night, having the urge of peeing more than six times. My sleeping time is not being bothered by my bladder problem anymore. I can also feel no tingling sensation, and it doesn't hurt to pee anymore.

# Chapter 8:
# The Restaurant

The history behind the man who loves to cook is pretty simple to tell. As the youngest of three boys, I am predictable, like other boys growing up in a small town. I am just an ordinary boy who loves the outdoors and sports and loves to cook.

My passion for cooking has been in my heart since I can't remember when. My mother used to say that if a man knows how to cook, he could rule the world. I used to be in the kitchen while my siblings played or did something like fixing my dad's motorcycle. Although I love sports and the outdoors, cooking is the best of them all.

It started with being the son who is always hungry. I used to help my mother around the kitchen to get things done immediately. My mother teaches me well, especially with all the ingredients and spices.

She, being half Italian, loves to serve and cook Italian dishes most of the time. We love her Bolognese and her Fettuccine. She can make the best Calzone and Ratatouille as well.

I told myself, I want to be like my mother. I want to cook for my wife and children someday. I will perfect all my sauces, and I will make my version of some Italian dishes and make it my signature dish.

And that's what happened when I had my own family. I made sure I cooked for them, and to add up, and I married the best woman and the best when it comes to desserts. We became the king and queen of our kitchen in the eyes of our children.

And now here I am, starting a new leaf in my life and beginning a fresh start after Margaret's death. I have proven to myself and my children that I am born solid and good in whatever endeavor I choose. With hard work and dedication, all my plans are in order.

The Idea of putting up a restaurant was when one of my friends suggested that I should travel or do something I love just to forget about Margaret's death for a while.

I was so devastated at that time, and my friends were there to cheer me up. They know that I am suffering deep inside and still hurting. When I heard about the suggestion, It suddenly crossed my mind.

It was a long-time dream for Margaret and me, and it was supposed to be our retirement plan. We are talking about it every night and were so excited to push through with that plan. We have been saving money for it and are very eager to pursue it at the right time.

When I mentioned it to Margaret, her face lightened up, and she said she had the same thought. She said we could pull it off because we both love to cook.

She said that she had had it in mind for some time now because We both agreed that I would retire early. We don't have any mortgage, and by the time the kids finish schooling, we will save money for the restaurant.

After Justin graduated from college, Margaret and I tried to save. She then accepted baking orders from close friends who loved her baked goodies. Her talent in baking kept us when we were aiming for financial stability.

Her enthusiasm inspires me to accept more projects to earn more money to pursue our dream. That's what I like about my wife. If she loves what she is doing, no one can stop her. It is like she doesn't get tired at all.

Every time we go to bed, we talk about it, dreaming of what it will be. Margaret said that we would look and buy a place near the beach that is very accessible to all prospective customers and the vast parking space to cater more.

I said that I would do the building design, and she would take care of the design. What Margaret touches, it always turns out to be beautiful. She can make simple things and turn them into exquisite ones.

When she got sick, all our dreams collided. All our savings were gone from the medications and chemotherapy. I haven't thought about it anymore because there is no point pursuing it for me.

I never thought that I could pursue this all alone. It takes many guts to have pushed it through. Thanks to my friends, the Idea came back, and I said to myself, "It's now or never."

Being in the dark after her death, the feeling of being lost and alone, I almost lost everything, including myself.

The restaurant has the best location in the city. I was so lucky to have found and bought that place. It was an old building but had many potentials, once a diner.

The owner sold this excellent place because he was too old to manage it. It was a little expensive due to the significant area, and the location itself is very accessible and very friendly. My money's worth having that place. The parking area is huge and very spacious. It is the best location for the restaurant.

Honestly, putting up the restaurant is not that hard for me. With the best motivation to be eager to cope with Margaret's death and the support of my loved ones, I did it very fast, unlike the others. The place has a minor renovation, and all the areas inside are what I would like it to be. It is like, it was arranged just for me.

Now, here it is, our long-time dream. I can see Margaret is smiling up there, feeling proud of what I did. The restaurant is operating and making people happy and satisfied.

All the people give good reviews and keep coming back. The location, the ambiance, the food, the coffee, and the people serving makes us the best place for Italian treats. We are growing faster, and people are waiting and lining up just to be done.

As we grow, there are several demands, but I stick to not having two or more outlets. We now have deliveries in some areas, and we have our website. Tanner designed it, and now some customers can download the app online and order very quickly.

The place now is jam-packed almost every weekend, and Jessie always thinks of having different promotions every month like having live bands at the parking area or promotions like buy one take one from all kinds of pizza. She always has the brightest ideas for promotions and always comes up with great views.

Now the restaurant is in great shape. I am so lucky to have a great staff. From five people when I opened, I now have twelve and counting. We also have regulars who seem to have lured many people too.

Well, it is all about the taste of the food and our special pasta. I am offering the best pizza in this area, and all my coffee is a best seller. I hate to brag, but It is a whole package.

Seeing that the business is good and helped me get through my problems is a win-win situation for my family and me. It is like, I am guided in the right path after Margaret's death.

The restaurant is my coping mechanism. My healer, my savior, the best decision.

Now seeing its success and running it gives me satisfaction and gives me the reason to get up every morning. I am happy with the outcome, and I am beginning to be financially stable again.

I am saying to myself that I couldn't ask for more. I just have to have faith in myself running this restaurant to be at its best. Continue to let it flourish and continue to give my customers satisfaction. "Maggie's Ristorante Italiano" will be at the top when the time comes. As for now, I am sharing my best efforts and heart with my business. It will be an honor to hand Margaret's and my legacy to our children and grandchildren.

# Chapter 9:
# The Lady in Red

It was a rainy Tuesday night with not a lot going on at the moment. I was sitting at the table near the door when somebody came in, and all I can say is, it has the most beautiful scent that captivates the air.

I immediately looked, wondering who it was, and I saw a lovely woman who glanced at me and gave me a timid smile that made me freeze for a moment. She was wearing a red dress. For the first time in a long time, I never have a single doubt that a woman will attract me again.

As she orders, I can hear the clarity of her calming voice, and as she smiles, I can see her perfect smile, which captivated me. I was stoned as if I am a statue at the moment that I overlooked that my youngest came into the door calling me, "Dad, are you okay?"

Justin was grinning at me because he noticed that I was staring at her. He said I wasn't blinking. She was so mesmerizing that until the moment she left the restaurant, I was just there sitting like a stupid fool. I went home and thought of her as a teenager.

The following day, I get up like I feel young and excited. I took a shower and went to the restaurant like I wanted to see her again. I tried to pull the time faster. I was waiting for her as if it were forever.

Every time the door opens, I bend over like a desperate guy. Sadly, she never showed up, and I felt so devastated not to see her that night. I went home sad and feeling like I had lost in a game. I never sleep well, thinking of her and having the discomfort of peeing now and then.

Two days passed by, and I never saw a glimpse of her. Then with all the customers around on a jam-packed night, one of my waiters asked if I could check on the newly arrived customers outside. It was a jam, so I hurriedly went out, not even thinking that the mystery woman was sitting at one of the tables outside.

My heart stopped seeing her, but I said to myself, this is it, I have a chance to approach her and get her order. When I ask her, "Hi, what can I get you?" She looked up and smiled, and then she said, "Can I have my usual coffee and a Tuna Pesto."

I was so confused by what she said, but don't have the guts to ask her again. Then the moment I walked on the counter I asked all of them about her and they all replied: "oh, she has been regular. She has been here every day since last month. That is her favorite spot, and she always orders a cup of cappuccino."

I am so stupid without knowing that she only went inside because It was raining that night. I never realized that she had been a constant customer for the past two years. I gathered information about her from my waiters. It is the best boss, and you get all the info you want!

I know that she works at the nearby library and is there almost every day except weekends—Mari,42, Mexican by blood, single, and very friendly. The best thing is that she loves all the meals that I offer. She has a favorite spot in my restaurant, and I am happy to know that.

The next day, it was raining again and at the same time when I first saw her, she came in. She was a vision in blue, my favorite color, by the way, as she approached one of the tables. I hurriedly went her way and took her to the table near the counter to see her clearly where I was stationed. I told her to try our new pizza flavor, and she agreed.

I did all the serving and went back and forth to check on her most of the time. My staff was smiling all the time, seeing me doing the serving. I am so eager to please her that I keep asking her what else she wants.

The next thing I know, I am sitting with her at the table talking to her, and it is so amusing because she is easy to talk to as if she knows me already. The night ended with an overwhelming feeling that I was eager to know her better.

After weeks of seeing and talking to her at the Restaurant, I played my cards well. Even though I hadn't done it in a long time, I finally took the courage to ask her out. Gladly she said yes. I said to myself, "Jeff, this is it. You can do it." I confide it to my friends, and they support me all the way.

"The day" has come. I am so eager to look as best as I can. I was so stressed and all because I wanted it to be perfect. As I was preparing, I was so nervous that I kept on going back and forth to the restroom peeing. I was looking dashing and tall, but the fact that my bladder was going nuts made me more anxious.

And then the truth just suddenly hit me, about how I have suffered for a long time and why I didn't do anything about it. Now, I am just crossing my fingers, hoping it will not bother us tonight.

A friend of mine let me borrow his yacht, and it was supposed to be a surprise because she only thought that we would have a little stroll on the beach and have a picnic later on.

As she approached my car, she looked divine, very stunning in pink. I am smiling at the back of my mind, realizing that I am very observant of Mari's details, like the color of her dresses. As she enters my car, the wind blows, and I can smell her perfume, the same scent that captivates me. The whole time we were on the way, she was so light that I forgot that I was so worried about my bladder.

As we are having a good time on the yacht, there it goes, my bladder is stealing the moment, our moment together. The third time I excused myself, Mari asked me if something was wrong. She was very persistent that I told her the truth. I told her that the peeing thing kept on bugging me lately. I told her that it started way back, but I have ignored it recently.

To my surprise, she too suffers from frequent Urinary Tract infections, and to add it up, the husband of her sister's best friend is a doctor. Excellent, we are meant to be. The day ended with me so comfortable talking about anything under the sun. And I agreed with her to see the doctor the next day.

As I walked her to the door, I had the urge to pee again, and I didn't want to destroy the moment and the excitement of our first kiss. And because of the discomfort that I am feeling, she notices my facial expression. She just reminded me about the appointment, and we ended up shaking hands.

The following events were the best days of my life. We are almost together every day for the whole week, accompanying me to the doctor's appointments. Even though we haven't kissed, I was so happy spending time with her and that I was diagnosed correctly with the proper medications like antibiotics.

She also encourages me to eat healthily, be hydrated, exercise, and take care of myself. She is good company at all times, and I thank her for convincing me to see her doctor.

I am delighted with the outcome of my appointment, plus the fact that being together makes it more beautiful because my feelings blossomed. Mari is also spending more time at the restaurant.

Even on weekends, she is there and what amazed me more was that she shows interest in what I love to do and keeps on watching me while cooking, which excites me more.

I can sense that she likes me too because she always hangs out at the Restaurant and never hesitates to give me a call to ask how my day is. After a week of medication, I can feel that I am feeling better because of no excessive feeling of going to the bathroom and peeing all the time.

Now, I want to ask her out again for the second time around, but I want it to be remarkable. I want to cook for her and show her how I work my magic in the kitchen and how my late wife fell in love with me because I cook the best meal.

I asked her out, and once again, she said yes. This time I invited her to my place. I was planning on giving her the best meal of her life and hoping that I would impress her this time.

The day came. I was so busy and preoccupied, and a lot was going on in my mind at that moment. I prepared a decent meal with the famous dessert I made for Margaret and the kids before. I hope this time it will impress her.

She is a vision of blue again and still smells that beautiful scent that catches my attention. We had the best talk during dinner, she told me everything I wanted to know about her, and as a librarian, she sure knows how to tell beautiful stories of her life like in the books. I became more interested in her as she confided her true-life story.

Her real name is Mari Felicia Martinez, 42 years old from Mexico. She emigrated to America at two with her parents, grandparents, and siblings. She has two sisters, and her mother was pregnant during that time.

Her parents decided to go to America because her father was offered a job, and it was for greener pastures because life in Mexico is not that great for them. Mari's father worked at a local library, and her mother made personalized pots to help her father earn money.

She is the eldest among her siblings. Mari loved to read books at a young age and was helping her mother with their little pottery business. She is the type of kid that is very responsible for her age. Mari is her mother's favorite because she can do everything, and she is brilliant as well.

As her grandparents were old and her mother was pregnant, she helped with cleaning, cooking, and laundry.

There were days that she could not do anything due to tiredness and lack of sleep because of all the things she was doing at a young age. But she always remembers her mother's words that you have to persevere through pain and diligence to achieve one's goal.

Mari's family was a Catholic, and she was one of the lucky children that were given a scholarship in a Catholic School that their church adopted. She is also a consistent honor student. As a keen reader, Mari is good at spelling and always a contestant in a spelling bee competition. She brings pride to their school by consistently winning the first prize.

Mari is a shy girl, but she grew up as a pleasant and well-spoken teenager and can speak well. She is becoming a beautiful young lady as well. Her teachers love her as well as her classmates—an up-and-coming young woman, to be exact.

As their little business grows, her father and mother consistently deliver orders from different states over the weekend. One Saturday morning, Mari's parents went upstate to deal with all their products, and sadly they got into a car accident that took away their lives. Mari was only thirteen years old at that time.

As her grandparents are getting older, being the most senior, Mari stands as the strongest because she is deciding at a very young age. The business is already gone, and they have to make ends meet with little savings that their parents left them. She is working in their church and studying at the same time.

Through her hard work and perseverance, she graduated and achieved excellent results and was honored and demanded from different high schools within the state and various state universities. As a keen reader, she is good at languages, so the local library hired her after graduation.

Outside her work, she was still that shy type of a woman who was having a hard time finding a date or going and meeting up with someone. It was a little hard to believe because she is very stunning and well, I can say that a head-turner. Of course, she got all the invitations from her workmates to go to a party, but she said she finds it hard to fit in because she is shy and unsure.

As a Mexican and a catholic, her upbringing is a little traditional and very conservative. As she was growing up, her grandparents were very strict that she has not been on a date ever since.

Meaning she never had a boyfriend since birth. Mari said that even though she is friendly and very articulate, if ever a guy is checking her out, she becomes too shy again to check him out too.

She told me her story, and I felt like I was glued to my seat because I was so interested in her life. It seems that I am beginning to like her more and more.

I also remember when my staff told me that when Mari started to dine in the restaurant, she loved being situated in a quiet place to read. And the team will look at her and be so amazed because of her gentleness if she is talking.

I have noticed some mannerisms in her ever since we started talking and dating, but now those mannerisms are even more visible because I know that she is comfortable talking to me.

Mari loves to touch her hair on her forehead when she is nervous and thinks of what else to say. She also loves to pout her lips if she is listening. And interested in the topic of the person is talking to her. But most of all, Mari has a beautiful tone if ever she is laughing hard.

I find interest in her life, and as Margaret, she also is a strong woman. She said she had been a regular in my restaurant for almost two years now, and it bugs me why I haven't laid my eyes on her in a long time. I was so preoccupied during those times and coping with Margaret's death and keeping the restaurant where it is right now.

One topic piques my interest of all the things we have to talk about that night. Mari said that she was a regular in the Mexican Restaurant before the library.

She was having a busy day and was very hungry, so she went there late in the afternoon to order some takeout. As she arrived at the counter to place her order, another person was giving his order too, and it made her turn back because he had the most admirable, soft voice similar to his dad.

The person next to the counter who took her and the gentleman's order made a mistake and gave them the wrong bags. Mari tried to take some food out of the bag as she left, but she realized it wasn't what she had ordered. She hurriedly went back to exchange her order, but sadly the gentleman had already left, taking her charge too.

She then told me that after six months, my restaurant opened and that her co-workers asked her to tag along to taste our food, and she loved it. From that day on, she sometimes passes by to order take out until the day that we put some tables and chairs outside and that she loves the view and picks her favorite spot. By that time, she always hangs out at my restaurant except on weekends because she likes to spend it with her family.

I was shocked, and I am that gentleman she referred to in her story. That day, I was looking for a place to put up my restaurant. I just passed by that Mexican Restaurant to get something to bite on my way home. I also was a little confused that time because I got the wrong order in the bag, and it's just too far to get back, so I just ate it anyway. I can do nothing because it is too late to get it back.

Now I remember where I had smelled that perfume before, and I love the scent of it. The woman next to me in that restaurant was Mari. I can still remember turning back at her, but she talked on her phone, so I didn't see her face. Although she smelled so good, I was in agony that time. It just slipped my mind.

I don't want that night to end, and I keep on holding on to every moment of it. Her personality is too different from Margaret's, and for me, it is a new start because Mari is so light and easy this time.

For the first time in a long time, I can say, and I am sure that I am totally into her and that I know that my children will like her. As I walked her towards her car, I trembled, telling myself, this is it! I don't know, but the feeling of being so intensely excited and nervous. I had never felt this way in a long time. Mari said that the meal was glorious and would look forward to another meal with me.

The moment has come. I grabbed Mari's hand and pulled her over next to me as we were saying goodbye. I looked at her beautiful eyes and gently brushed my lips towards hers. It was only a minute, but it felt like it was the most extended kiss I have ever had in a long time.

It was a blast, and the next day I was so happy that I called my kids to meet me for lunch in the restaurant. I made their favorite Calzone and their favorite pizza. While we were eating, I told them about the girl who made me smile again. I never expected their reaction because I was a little bit worried that they might have a violent response.

They love their mother so much that they mourn like me for a very long time. It was exciting because Jessie said, "give us the details, dad!" She was so eager to know how we met. On the other hand, Justin suggested that I invite her to his place over the weekend, and he convinced me to bring Mari so that they could meet her.

So, this is it, my children accept that I am dating again, and I am delighted to know that they are very open that I will soon be in a relationship again.

Mari and I have a good time going to my son's house in the car. Although I can feel her tense that she will meet my children for the first time, she is taking it lightly, which I like about her. She is being cool while holding my hand.

When we arrived, I could sense that my children were very eager to meet her. The reaction on their faces is apparent that they want to see if my description was fitting.

My children were giving me a thumbs up, and I knew from that very moment that they liked her. Even my grandchildren adore her. As we are having dinner, the discussion is very flowing, and they are talking as if they already knew each other. We left with a light feeling in my heart that they all accepted her.

The next day my daughter called me and told me that they were happy that I was well and seeing someone. She said that Justin likes Mari as she does. As they met and were introduced, she said they felt and saw a certain resemblance to their late mother.

I was shocked, and I never thought they saw her that way. Maybe they are right because even though I can't see it yet, how she captivates me is like how Margaret did. I went to sleep that night thinking about what my life would be like without Mari in it. I know that I love Margaret dearly deep in my heart, but this is something new to me after a long time.

I am me again. I am a man who loves life to the fullest and wants to explore again. I feel young and singing in the shower again. My children are very welcome to the Idea of it, which makes me feel confident that everything will be okay.

If I turn back, I am in the dark for the longest time, and I can't imagine my life if I stayed in that dark as long as I can imagine. It's been four years that I have been coping and healing. I may not be as great as I was, but I know that I am in great shape now when Margaret died.

"The Lady in Red" came into my life and caught my attention. I never expected this, and I never thought I would fall in love again. Mari is my future, and I cannot deny it anymore. She brings out the best in me again after a long time. Now I am sure that I want to spend the following years of my life with her.

After almost nine months of dating and knowing Mari, I finally realized that I couldn't stand not seeing her every day. She made me happy, and I think it's about time to decide to propose. I ask my children for blessings and tell them that I am sure that I want her in my life.

Jessie said they want me to be happy and are sure that their mother would like that. My friends are willing to help me find a romantic way to pop the big question to her. They all agree with my decision and suggest many ways for this exciting event. I was set to pop the question on a Tuesday night, and everybody was invited and excited.

It has been a roller coaster ride for almost a year, and my Restaurant is doing great. I have experienced my bladder infection and was cured. I never imagined dating again and, most of all, being in love again.

I thought that life was tied to my Restaurant, still moving on from Margaret's death, being a father and a mother to my children, being the best grandad to my grandchildren, and dealing with old age. Until the day that Mari came into my life.

I suffered in pain when my wife died, and I thought I could never return to my old self again. Having problems with my Bladder also bugs me because it gives me discomfort. The moment of truth is here. Everybody is around and excited. The place looks fantastic as we have been waiting for Mari for almost an hour now. The more I wait, the more anxious I become more excited.

Mari never showed up that evening. I was so worried that I kept calling her, but she never answered her phone. My children were concerned too, and Jessie, like herself, found a way to know where Mari was until Mari found the number of Mari's sister. She then called and found that Mari was rushed to the hospital early that afternoon.

My kids and I then went to the hospital as fast as we could, and there she was, admitted for further observation. I talked to the Doctor, and He said that She was vomiting, had a high fever, and was having chills. Acute Urinary Tract Infection is the findings.

# Chapter 10:
# Mari's Problem

Mari, as being shy, usually keeps everything to herself. She also doesn't want anybody to be worried for her. As being the eldest, her siblings are her priority. She was the tough one in her family, and she saw to it that her family was always in good hands.

Working hard and taking all the responsibility is her aim, but sadly she forgot about herself. She is the type to put her loved ones and others before her. She always takes herself for granted.

Taking care of herself is always not a priority to her. Being busy and working long hours is Mari's usual routine. Mari also suffers from bladder problems because of the urge to urinate if she is active and not taking good care of herself most of the time.

The recurrence of her UTI is the reason why she was hospitalized. She kept on neglecting the thought that she was feeling something. I never thought that she had a fever and discomfort. She doesn't look sick if she is with me. However, I have noticed that she always excuses herself to go to the bathroom most of the time.

The doctors said she might be experiencing symptoms again, but she is getting used to it because she feels that way. Mari is very prone to recurrence as a busy person and a workaholic. She has a low Immune system, too, said the doctor.

I never left her side the whole time. Mari was there for me and convinced me when I was the one who was suffering. I volunteered to watch over her, and my children agreed and took care of the restaurant while I was away. I want her to see my face at the moment. She opens her eyes. I will never leave the woman I loved.

Mari stayed in the hospital for three days, and she is in progress as usual. She is a fighter. With the proper medication, Mari gets well that fast. I know that she is powerful. She is just the type of person that puts the welfare of others first than herself.

Mari has an overactive bladder, and she is very sickly too. She often gets embarrassed because her condition pushes her to urinate uncontrollably, so she has to wear napkins or diapers whenever we go out or even if we stay home.

During our stay in the hospital, the doctors would require her not to use diapers all the time. So, she would often wake up many times in the middle of the night because she urges to urinate. She would quietly find her way to the restroom, worrying that she would disturb my sleep. But I wouldn't want her to feel like she's on her own, so I would pretend that I woke up too.

Then, after she goes out of the restroom, I would prepare a cup of tea or some crackers for her, explaining how hospitals make me feel hungry all the time, and we would laugh about it until she fell back to sleep.

It's funny because I would love to look at her while sleeping. I wonder why such a beautiful person is still alone and not married. And then, I would say to myself, she is waiting for me and just smile inside until I fall asleep again.

Mari is capturing my heart more and more every single day. The way she smiles when I hand her favorite cup of coffee, the way she peacefully curves her lips when she's fast asleep, and the way she dances when she's finally getting her tummy filled with food. And the best part is every time. She says thank you to me while touching my shoulders.

When the time came that the doctor had discharged Mari, I immediately asked if I could let her use Flotrol too. He just smiled and tapped me on my shoulder, saying, "Hey, if it works for both of us, I am sure it will work for her too!" "Don't you worry, my wife is a number fan of Flotrol," then he winks at me.

I brought her home and planned to stay with her for a few days. I know she will never be comfortable in my apartment, so I decided to make her comfortable in her own home.

When Jessie and Tanner arrived, I hurriedly back home to get my things and my bladder supplement "Flotrol "so that Mari could try it too. I hope it will work for her never to be bothered by her bladder problems again.

I arrived, and I was so amazed seeing that my daughter was cooking for Mari. She made her mashed potato, pork ribs steak, and caesar's salad. Tanner bought all the ingredients at the nearby store.

It took a while before going back since I passed by the restaurant to get some elements too because I plan to prepare her a nice dinner. Patricia rocks taking care of the restaurant while I was gone and busy taking care of Mari.

That's family for me, and they always got each other's back. And now I am happy that they consider Mari as one too. Jessie was so delightful that evening. Cooking for Mari and saying that she would bring Mari's laundry to the shop while Tanner was the one who did the dishes that night.

I am so thankful that they all like her and are very concerned about her welfare. Mari is so appreciative to Jessie and Tanner and keeps saying thank you, Jessie just winked at her saying, "Hey, we got you. "

That night, I put Mari to sleep and just watched her, imagining what would be our life together. I planned to propose to her that night, and now I must find the right time again. I stayed with her for three days and let her try Flotrol, and I was crossing my fingers that it would work for her.

I promise myself that I will take care of Mari from now on. She took care of me when I had my recurrence, and now it is my turn to do the same. Currently, Mari is becoming a part of me, making me happy.

I never thought that I would feel like this again after Margaret died. I thought I would be that widower who will spend the rest of his life feeling miserable and sad toward the passing of his late wife. But the moment I saw Mari, that thought vanished into thin air.

I am determined that this woman will make me so happy again. So, whatever happens, I won't leave her side. She is the reason for my smile and my strength. I am not going to throw away my second chance at happiness. That is why I promised myself that I would be substantial, not only for me but for Mari too.

# Chapter 11:
# Getting to Know

Aging is like forgetting some things you do when you are still young. Courting a girl, for instance, or going to dates and impressing them. Worst case for me because I only courted one girl, and I married her. I thought that love would last a lifetime.

Sadly, it wasn't the case for me because the love of my life left me very early.

But as the famous saying goes, there will always be a rainbow after the rain. After years of being alone, I never thought that a woman would capture my attention again. Of course, no one can be compared to Margaret, and she is one of a kind.

However, Mari is unique, too, in her ways. She has a very light personality, easy to deal with, and is a fun company to have. She is fantastic, like a breath of fresh air.

I am very much interested in getting to know her better. I am very captivated by her on all levels. Her looks, smile, scent, light attitude, and way she appreciates little things. The fact that she excites me is very unusual but very interesting. To sum it up, Mari is a woman I long for in my life now.

She is the woman I never thought I needed, and she came into my life at the right time. I can see it now, Margaret was my first love, but Mari will be my savior, the one who made my heartbeat again after it died together with my first love. Mari was the love that I needed, and I will do whatever it takes to let her realize how we are meant for each other.

I know that having a bladder problem is irritating and not good, but I somehow thank it because I got the chance to get to know Mari better. Spending time with her during doctor's appointments and the thought that she convinced me to see a doctor is astounding. Even Margaret and my children are always having a hard time saying yes unless I am sure for myself.

But Mari had this power over me, and I'm not viewing this as unfavorable. This power she had excites me because it makes me do things I haven't done before, and one thing is it pushes me to take the time to take care of myself.

Mari was very comfortable with me when she had opened up about her life. Telling me all the details makes me wonder, how can a beautiful creature suffer at an early age and not be so sure about herself despite all the achievements and honors during her schooldays?

She doesn't see herself as beautiful as she is. She didn't know how amazing she was, and as I got to know her better, the more I fell for her. All the things that I learned about her made me feel giddy and excited because she is so ignorant of how beautiful she is as a person.

There are days when I would tease her and tell her that if only, I had the power to pluck out my eyes and lend them to her so that she could see herself the way I see her, I would do it in a heartbeat. If she would laugh intensely and loudly while patting my shoulders, and that right there was another perfect moment encrypted in my memory.

She has the perfect laugh. So crisp and very inviting. Sometimes hearing it makes me shiver because Margaret laughs like that too. It is like the two women that made me fall in love have the most beautiful sound when they laugh.

I'm not asking for much. That is why I grabbed each chance to spend time with Mari. It may be a simple lunch date or a couple of checkups; sign me in. I am good if I get to spend some quality time with her.

Knowing her is like the best second chance I got. So, I want to preserve each memory together, whether something out of the blue or something completely unexpected. Mari and I will write forever, one step at a time.

# Chapter 12:
# I Was Healed by Flotrol

I am glad that I have taken the Flotrol Natural Bladder Support Supplement. I know that I haven't been good to my body all those years. I had neglected myself, especially when Margaret was sick. Worst of all, I engaged in vices like drinking and smoking after She died. I could not blame it on anyone else but me.

When Mari came into my life, I experienced embarrassment during our first date. I have been experiencing symptoms again, but I keep on ignoring it until the day that I can no longer hold my pee. I was so embarrassed about what happened to me, and I thought that was the end of my love life, but gladly, it became the way of a new beginning with Mari.

I know that I should have avoided those kinds of moments by searching for good remedies online or asking and listening to some friend's advice, but I became so stubborn that I only listened to myself. Now, I am more aware of the damage if I take it for granted.

With all the natural ingredients that Flotrol offers, it is very safe to use it. Research shows that relief varies for different kinds of people. Some have excellent results right away, and some can feel relief after a week. On my part, I think that it worked for me after three days of consistent usage.

Flotrol is clinically proven with very safe ingredients that many can trust. It contains pumpkin seeds and soy extracts proven to heal bladder problems during the olden days. It is specially formulated for mature people to cure bladder problems.

It is easy to swallow, makes it easy for you to take it, and is very convenient to those who would like to purchase it online. No prescription is needed.

I am relieved of all the sleepless nights and discomfort because of the Flotrol Natural Bladder Support Supplement. I am glad to have used this product, and I can willingly attest to the product.

It worked for me, and it might as well work for you. No worries to those suffering from discomfort, pain, and embarrassment due to bladder problems; Flotrol can change that and let it all disappear.

With the help of Flotrol, I am delighted with the results. Now I am experiencing my life to the fullest. A widower, A father, A grandfather, an engineer turned entrepreneur, A man who is at his prime and in love with a beautiful woman. I am enjoying life that is so beautiful with my family and Mari.

I never experienced side effects with its natural ingredients, unlike the anti-biotics I was using before. If only I had taken this product earlier, I know that I might not have the recurrence, and maybe I enjoyed my first date with Mari.

Now I recommend it to Mari and my friends who have trouble with their bladder. I am sure that they will have the relief that the product gave me. Mari has been using the product for almost a month now, and She is also happy with the results.

We are delighted to use the product and enjoy the promo they offer. We are pleased with the results and very much to have our money's worth spending. Like us, you too can enjoy your life again without a bladder problem. It worked for us, and I am sure It will work for you too.

You can purchase it at the convenience of your home or wherever you are. It is effortless to buy it by using your laptop or your phone. All you have to do is go to their website and click. It will be delivered to your doorstep, and it's hassle-free because there is no need for you to go out, and the best part is that you don't need a prescription to buy it.

Flotrol is life-changing. I am confident to say goodbye to sleepless nights, frequent trips to the toilet, pain, discomfort, embarrassment. I am free of it and very much happier now. I now can sleep well, eat well, feel healthier, and most of all enjoy my life to the fullest by spending it with my loved ones. I travel long trips without worries and anxiety.

Taking care of ourselves is a must. We have to be aware of what's going on in our bodies. We must not neglect any signs and symptoms that we are experiencing. We are the owner of our bodies, and we must take care of them. Always remember that prevention is better than cure. We owe ourselves to be taken care of most of the time. After all, we have only one life to live.

With a healthy lifestyle like exercising, eating healthy food, keeping hydrated all the time, sleeping well, and taking Flotrol, I assure you, you will be happier and healthier. Imagine a life of worry-free bladder problems, a life worth living. As the saying goes, "Don't let your age stop you from doing everything. " So, we all know that age is one of the reasons why we have bladder problems.

So don't let your bladder control your life, act now, do it now. Take Flotrol and be amazed by its results. Take it from a guy who used it every day. I tell it's a money-back guarantee and worth trying.

# Chapter 13:
# What is Urinary Tract Health?

The Urinary Tract comprises kidneys, the bladder, and the tubes leading to and from these organs. The Ureters and the Urethra produce urine and eliminate it from the body.

Urine goes from the kidneys to the bladder for storage through two tubes called the Urethra, which create urine while filtering waste items from the blood. In females, it opens in front of the vagina, while in men, it opens at the tip of the penis.

The health of the urinary tract refers to how well the system removes wastes, generates, and manages urine and any illnesses or abnormalities that may occur inside the tract. These issues can affect the entire urinary tract or just certain parts, such as the bladder.

This section focuses on two more common disorders related to urinary tract health for women: Urinary Tract Infection (UTI) and Urinary Incontinence (UI).

1) Urinary Tract Infection (UTI)- is a common infection, usually caused by bacteria in the bladder or Urethra.

There are several kinds of UTI. The type of this UTI depends on where the condition occurs.

- Urethritis- is an infection that happens in the Urethra of an individual.
- Cystitis- is an infection that occurs in the bladder.

A UTI can spread up one or both ureters to the kidney, causing pyelonephritis or kidney infection if left untreated. It can progress to the point where hospitalization is required as part of treatment. Kidney infection is more common in women than males, and UTIs are not the primary cause. They can also have an impact on youngsters.

2) Urinary incontinence, also known as UI, is another bladder condition. This condition describes the loss of bladder control

or inability of an individual to control their micturition.

UI can affect all individuals in society. Men, women, and children are more likely to experience UI than men because of their female urinary tract structure and the effects of pregnancy, childbirth, and menopause. UI is also common among older women, although it is not typical for aging people.

- Stress incontinence is frequently caused by structural problems, such as the bladder not being correctly positioned. Urine leaks might happen whether you're laughing, coughing, exercising, lifting, or doing nothing at all.
- Urge incontinence, often known as overactive bladder, is caused by a muscle that surrounds the bladder. It occurs when urine escapes at inconvenient times, such as when sleeping. Urge incontinence is more common in older people and isn't always a sign of a urinary tract infection. It's also linked to neurological diseases like multiple sclerosis.
- Overflow Incontinence occurs when a bladder is overfilled and urine leaks uncontrollably. Overflow incontinence causes a person to feel unable to empty their bladder. Tumors, kidney stones, diabetes, and drugs are some causes. Men are the ones who have it the most.
- Functional incontinence is the inability to use the restroom on time due to a physical or other impairment.
- Mixed incontinence occurs when a person has more than one form of incontinence, such as stress and urge incontinence.
- Transient incontinence occurs when urine leaking is triggered by a transitory condition such as an infection or new medicine. When the source of the contradiction is removed, the inconsistency vanishes.

# Chapter 14:
# Bladder Infection

Bladder infections have a way of drawing your attention to focus on it. You will try many going to the bathroom, yet you will still feel the need to pee. When you urinate, you may have discomfort and a burning feeling. This is an early symptom that you have a bladder infection.

When you have a bladder infection, it causes cystitis, when your bladder swells and becomes irritable. That is what is causing your symptoms and suffering. The most frequent type of Urinary Tract Infection is a bladder infection.

Here are the main parts of the urinary tract system and its function:

- Kidneys- clean the waste from your blood and make you pee regularly.
- Ureters- are two thin tubes, one for each kidney. It then carries pee directly to your bladder.
- Bladder- is responsible for storing your pee.
- Urethra- carries pee from the bladder to outside your body.

Women are more prone to get bladder infections than men. Usually, the condition is more annoying than serious, and antibiotics are the treatment. If untreated, it can travel up to the ureters and the kidneys and cause severe problems.

Having a weakened immune system or a chronic health condition can increase your susceptibility to repeated infections, including UTIs. Diabetes, together with other autoimmune disorders, neurological diseases, and kidney or bladder stones, raises your UTI risk.

Unless you are fortunate enough to have never had a UTI, you will never be aware of its symptoms. Thirty percent of women who have had a urinary tract infection had a recurrence within six months.

If you've had multiple UTIs, you've seen the toll they take on your life. However, you can take solace in knowing that they aren't the product of anything you've done. Recurrent UTIs aren't caused by inadequate cleanliness or anything else that women have done to themselves. Some women are predisposed to UTIs.

# Chapter 15:
# What are the Causes?

As people age, health changes and problems in your bladder occur. Bladder problems and UTI are very common to men and women at a certain age. It has been proven that bladder problems can massively affect your quality of life. Lifestyle can also be one of the main reasons you will experience this kind of problem.

The bladder is identified as the hollow organ found in the lower abdomen, where pee is stored. As the bladder fills, the muscles in its wall relax, allowing it to expand.

As the bladder empties during urination, the muscles also contract and force the pee out via the urethra. A variety of bladder issues can cause pain.

These are the three most common causes of pain.

- Interstitial cystitis is a poorly known bladder illness that causes chronic pelvic pain and urination difficulties. It's also known as bladder discomfort syndrome or painful bladder syndrome. The condition primarily affects adults in their 30s and 40s, and it affects both men and women equally.
- Urinary tract infection (UTI) is an illness that can affect any part of your urinary system, including your kidneys, ureters, bladder, and urethra. It is helpful to know that the bladder and urethra, located in the lower urinary system, are involved in most illnesses. But even if that is the case, UTI is still more common in women than in men. A bladder infection can be highly inconvenient. A UTI that spreads to your kidneys, on the other hand, could have serious consequences.
- Bladder Cancer is a form of cancer that starts in the bladder cells. Bladder cancer usually begins in the cells that line the lining of your bladder (urothelial cells). Your kidneys and the tubes (ureters) that connect the kidneys and the bladder also contain urothelial cells. It can occur in the kidneys and ureters, although it is more likely to happen in the bladder.

Bacteria, generally E. coli, are the main culprits. Coli. These bacteria can be found on your skin and in your intestines, and they're usually harmless. They're all around us. They can sneak into the urethra in various ways and end up in the bladder, causing infection. Prostate infections are the most common cause of them in males. Even yet, any obstruction, such as a bladder stone or an enlarged prostate, might prevent the bladder from emptying, resulting in illness. However, women have many chances to get them due to their urethra being shorter than men. It is close to the vagina and anus, where the bacteria live. `

Here are some common reasons in women that can cause this kind of problem.

- Having sex is very important to take care of your hygiene before and after sex. It is to avoid any bacteria that can cause UTI or other infections. Adding to it, you must pay attention to your partner; sexual intercourse may lead to cystitis, but you don't have to be active to develop it.
- Tampon- women have their regular period every month. Some use tampons, and some use napkins. It is a common cause of infection, especially if it has been worn too long. To avoid infections, you must make sure to change every hour during your period and always wash with water now and then, especially on your heavy days.
- Using diaphragm or birth control pills- using this method of birth control is risky sometimes. It has its disadvantages. Women using it are prone to bladder problems and other infections.
- Pregnancy: Pregnant women are prone to infection, and mostly, it is urinary tract infections.
- Menopause- women in their menopause have the most risk of having bladder problems and urinary tract infections. Changes in hormones can trigger a low immune system that can highly reason to acquire bladder problems.
- The acidity of urine. A new study shows that small molecules related to the diet may influence how well bacteria can grow in the urinary tract.

- Stress: UTI can be induced by stress. Feeling stressed is not a direct cause but leads to high cortisol levels, which reduces the effect on the immune system.
- Kidney stones- People with a blockage in their urinary tract, such as kidney stones, are more likely to get UTIs. An enlarged prostate gland of a man can also block the flow of urine and can cause a bladder infection.

There are so many reasons that can cause the bladder to be irritated. As we age, we develop weaknesses in our immune system that can trigger it. We are most likely prone to it, especially if we are not careful of eating.

Certain foods and beverages that can irritate the bladder, here are the most common:

- Caffeine can encourage the development of a UTI, but it does not cause it. Because caffeine is a diuretic, frequent urination causes dehydration in the body. During chronic dehydration, the urine reaches excessive salt concentrations, irritating the bladder.
- Alcohol can make you urinate more frequently. Alcohol's dehydrating effect may induce bladder irritation, such as pain and burning when peeing.
- Acidic fruits, such as oranges, grapefruits, lemons, and limes, as well as fruit drinks, might exacerbate bladder infection symptoms. Fruit is an integral part of a healthy diet. However, fruit that contains many acids can irritate and increase your UTI symptoms.
- Spicy foods should be avoided. If you have bladder infection symptoms, you should avoid them because they may irritate your bladder or worsen UTI systems.
- Avoid eating tomato-based products if you are experiencing any indications or symptoms of a bladder infection. Your UTI may be triggered or worsened by the acid.
- Carbonated drinks like citrus-flavored and carbonated sodas are known to exacerbate the symptoms of urinary tract infections. So, if you're having trouble with your bladder, you should stick to water.

- Chocolate has too much sugar can cause urinary tract infections since the germs that cause them to love sugar. It raises the acidity of your urine, hastening the progression of the illness.

# Chapter 16:
# What are the Signs and Symptoms?

Men and women all over the world often suffer from bladder infections. It is more often annoying than serious. They can travel up your kidneys, where they can cause more severe problems.

Some men and women feel discomfort, but some don't have any that they never realized that they have one. Each type of UTI may result in one or more signs and symptoms; it depends whether which part of the urinary tract is severely infected.

Here are some symptoms to watch for:

A robust and continuous urge to urinate and more peeing than average is hugely concerning.

It's not good when it wakes you up at least 20 times in the middle of the night.

You have a bladder infection. That's all it means.

When urinating, you may experience a scorching feeling different from dull, stabbing, or painful pain.

They were passing frequent tiny volumes of urine. If a person needs to pee regularly, but only a little bit comes out when they try, it could be related to UTI.

The urine appears to be cloudy. If the urine is yellowish in color than the usual clear, it could be alarming infections such as UTI or kidney stones.

Pee that smells like solid urine: Urine that smells like reliable urine is a typical side effect of UTIs. It's due to the germs found in the urine.

Pelvic discomfort affects women primarily in the lower abdomen. The pain could be constant or intermittent.

How do you know that you have a bladder infection? If you pee at least ten times in two hours, you might be wondering if you have a bladder infection. And well, you may be right, especially if it hurts, burns, or stings when you pee.

If you are experiencing lower back pain in your belly and having pee way more often than usual, you have a bladder infection or UTI.

# Chapter 17:
# The Risk Factors

Urinary tract infections are common to women, and many women experience more than one infection during a lifetime. It is riskier to women than to men.

Urinary tract abnormalities: Some babies are born with urinary tract abnormalities that don't allow urine to leave the body usually or cause the urine to back up in the urethra can increase the cause of UTI.

Blockages in the urinary tract- kidney stones or an enlarged prostate can trap urine in the bladder and increase UTI risk.

A suppressed immune system- Diabetes and other diseases that impair the immune system- the body's defense against germs- can increase the risk of bladder problems.

Catheter use- most men and women who can't urinate independently and use a tube (catheter) to urinate are at a greater risk for UTIs most of the time. It may include hospitalized people, people with neurological problems that make it difficult to control their urination ability and paralyzed people.

A recent urinary procedure, such as surgery or a medically assisted examination of your urinary tract can both raise your chance of developing a urinary tract infection.

People who acquire bladder infections treated immediately and adequately have lower risks of any complications. But if left untreated may suffer from tremendous and severe consequences.

Complications of UTI may include:

- Recurrent infections- this happens a lot to women who experience two or more UTIs in the span of six months or more within a year.
- Permanent kidney damage: The acute, chronic kidney infection (pyelonephritis) is primarily due to an untreated UTI. It can cause more damage to your health.

- Increased risk in pregnant women can cause a greater risk of giving birth to low birth weight or premature infants.
- Urethral narrowing (stricture)- in men from recurrent urethritis, previously seen with gonococcal urethritis.
- Sepsis is a potentially fatal infection consequence that occurs when an infection spreads from your intestines to your urinary tract and kidneys.

You have to feel your body, and bladder infection can be crucial, especially untreated. Always ask for medical help at once, most importantly if it hurts when you pee and if you have any of these signs that it only means then that you have a severe infection:

- Vomiting: Another more severe kind of UTI is an infection in your kidney. It causes you to vomit, so you must seek medical help.
- Fever: High fever is one common sign that you have a severe infection.
- Chills: It is a sign that you have high fever due to the bacteria causing the infection.
- Bloody urine: UTI can cause bloody urine. It is also called Hematuria.

Belly or back pain- UTIs typically cause bladder-specific symptoms like cloudy urine or pain when you urinate. It can affect your abdomen and trigger pain in your belly or back.

It may mean potentially life-threatening kidney disease, a prostate infection, a bladder or kidney tumor, or a urinary tract stone. You have to be aware of what's going on in your body. Here is some standard information that needs to be taken seriously:

1) Symptoms return after you've finished treatment.
2) You also have been discharged from your vagina or penis. It may be a sign of a sexually transmitted disease, pelvic inflammatory disease, or other severe infection.
3) You have ongoing pain or a hard time peeing. It may also be a sign of an STD, vaginal infection, kidney stone, enlargement of the prostate, or a bladder and prostate tumor. Or it could be that the disease is resistant to the Antibiotic your doctor

prescribes.

Getting checked if you feel something odd in your bladder or urine or if you have any signs and symptoms, is the best way. Seeking professional help is the best way to do it. There are medical ways to find out if there is something wrong.

Here are some examples of Diagnosis, Tests, and Procedures used to find out if you have a UTI:

Analyzing a urine sample- your doctor may ask for a urine sample for lab analysis to look for white blood cells or bacteria. To avoid potential sample contamination, you are advised to wash your feminine area before collecting the urine sample.

Growing bacteria in the urinary system in a lab- A urine culture is commonly performed after a lab urine analysis. This test will inform your doctor which germs are causing your infection and which drugs will work best.

An ultrasound, a computed tomography (CT) scan, or magnetic resonance imaging may be used to create illustrations of your urinary tract system if you have frequent infections that an abnormality in your urinary tract causes your doctor suspects. Your doctor may also use a contrast dye to highlight structures in your urinary tract.

If you have recurrent UTIs, your doctor may do a cystoscopy, which involves inserting a long thin tube with a lens into your urethra and bladder to examine the insides. The cystoscope is introduced into your urethra and your bladder.

**Risk factors that can make you prone to UTIs**

- Being a woman can make you more prone to having UTIs.
- A shorter gap between the anus and the urethra (the opening where urine exits the body)
- Having a history of urinary tract infections (especially in the past 12 months)
- Having a mother who has had urinary tract infections (UTIs)
- Having problems with your urinary tract (such as kidney stones)
- If you're a woman who's gone through menopause (due to

changes to the microorganisms in the vaginal area)

- If you have chronic conditions like Diabetes.
- In the last year, you've had new sexual partners.
- Having recently or frequently engaged in sexual activity
- Having recent or frequent sexual intercourse.
- I was not urinating before or after sexual intercourse.
- Using spermicide or spermicide-coated condoms.
- Using a diaphragm during intercourse.
- Wearing non-cotton underwear.

Bacteria can be found on the inside and outside of the human body. A UTI, on the other hand, can develop when bacteria from the gut or the skin migrate up the urethra and into the bladder, where they grow and cause infection. E. The most frequent bacteria that cause UTIs is E. coli, which is commonly detected.

No matter what they do, some women are more prone to UTIs. Some of the most effective preventative measures, on the other hand, are pretty easy. You must follow your doctor's instructions and take care of yourself.

Here are some nursing tips that can help you prevent UTI;

- Assess the symptoms of UTI.
- Please encourage them to drink at least eight glasses of water or healthy fluid.
- Administer antibiotics as ordered by your doctor.
- Encourage the patient to void frequently.
- Educate patients on proper wiping.
- Educate patients on drinking juices rich in vitamin c, which help the growth of bacteria.
- Please take the right antibiotics prescribed by your doctor, and do not skip them.

The risk of having can be prevented if you only follow your doctor's advice. The medicines you are taking can cure it and give you a remedy. Avoiding the risk is better because you will prevent more significant complications.

# Chapter 18:
# Home Remedies

As the saying goes, prevention is better than cure. You can either be careful of your health or you can take steps to reduce your risk of urinary tract infections. Taking care of yourself and taking precautions are very important. There are so many ways that we can prevent this problem from occurring.

Here are some simple ways that we can do at home for prevention;

- Drink plenty of fluids, especially water- drinking water helps dilute your urine and ensures that you'll urinate more frequently - allowing bacteria to be flushed from your urinary tract before an infection can begin.
- Drink cranberry juice- Although studies are not conclusive that cranberry juice prevents UTIs, it is likely, not harmful.
- Wipe from front to back- doing so after urinating and after a bowel movement helps prevent bacteria in the anal region from spreading to the vagina and urethra.
- Empty your bladder soon after intercourse- urinating after having sex is very healthy. Drinking a glass of water after sex so that you can pee, helps flush bacteria.
- Avoid potentially irritating feminine products- using deodorant sprays or other feminine products such as douches and powders, in the genital area can irritate the urethra.
- Change your birth control method- diaphragms, or unlubricated or spermicide-treated condoms, can all contribute to bacterial growth. It is also known as harmful to your health.

In order to practice self-care. Here are some things you can do at home to get relief;

- Avoid having sex.
- Drink lots of water and avoid alcohol, caffeine, spicy foods that can make your symptoms worse.
- Take a pain reliever.

- Try a 15- to 20-minute soak in a warm bath.
- Use a heating pad on your lower belly.

Getting a bladder infection once in a while may be a bother, but it's not usually a serious health concern. Sometimes, though, it's important to know the cause of the infection, because the medicine alone may not be enough to treat it.

Your doctor will first do a physical exam and talk to you about your symptoms. That may be enough to find out whether you have one. You then get your urine analyzed.

This is to determine if there is a bacteria present, blood, or worst pus in the sample of your pee. Your doctor will also run a urine culture to find out which bacteria are causing your infections.

As your doctor gives you the right medication you will feel relief but it does not stop there. You have to take care of yourself, eat the right kind of food, exercise regularly and you must avoid food and beverages that trigger your UTI.

It is also a must that you must not hold your urge to pee. Never hold it, always make sure that you empty your bladder so that it will not cause more complications.

You can also ease the pain you are suffering by taking a pain reliever. If you are experiencing pain due to a urinary tract infection, the following may help ease it.

Here are some tips to ease what you feel;

- Wear loose clothing- wearing loose clothing, preferably made from cotton or other natural materials will help keep moisture at bay and will keep moisture at bay and will make you feel more comfortable.
- Apply heat- use a heating pad, a warm washcloth, or a hot water bottle to apply heat to your bladder or pelvic area if you are feeling pain or discomfort from your UTI.
- Take a warm bath- there are some people who take a warm bath if ever they feel pain or discomfort. It helps them relax or helps their muscles relax.
- Take over-the-counter pain reliever- you can buy and use

medication that you can buy over the counter. Use caution here, always ask for professional help to avoid any kidney complications.

Always be aware of what you are feeling. You will know if there is something wrong with your body. Knowledge is always the key and the greater you are well informed, the better. Be cautious of your health and take good care of your body. We only have one life, and we owe it to ourselves.

# Chapter 19:
# Treatments

A visit to a doctor if you have the signs and the symptoms of UTI is the best thing to do. You must take the proper tests so that you can be properly diagnosed.

You can tell your doctor everything, like being allergic to medicines in your previous checkups. Telling him all your concerns and worries is also crucial; your doctor must know your history to prescribe you the best medication that can cure you.

Here are some examples of Antibiotic that gets rid of UTI the fastest;

1) Sulfamethoxazole/Trimethoprim (Bactrim)- is always the first choice because it works very well and can treat UTI in as fast as three days when you take it twice a day.
2) Nitrofurantoin (Macrobid)- is another first choice for UTIs, but it has to be taken longer than Bactrim.
3) Fosfomycin (Monurol)- is an antibiotic primarily used to treat lower UTI. Occasionally it is used for prostate infections. It is generally taken by mouth. However, there are some side effects, including diarrhea, nausea, headache, and vaginal yeast infections.
4) Cephalexin (Keflex)-is an antibiotic commonly used to treat bacterial infections, such as pneumonia, chest infections, and urinary tract infections.
5) Ceftriaxone- is an antibiotic used to treat many kinds of bacterial infections, including severe or life-threatening forms such as E. coli, pneumonia, or meningitis.
6) Ciprofloxacin- is a fluoroquinolone antibiotic used to treat several bacterial infections. It includes certain types of infectious diarrhea, respiratory tract infection, and urinary tract infection.
7) Levofloxacin- sold under the brand name of Levaquin, among others, it is an antibiotic used to treat different kinds of infection, including UTI.

8) Amoxicillin- It is most often used to treat several bacterial infections. It primarily includes middle ear infections, strep throat, Pneumonia, skin infections, and Urinary Tract Infections, among others. It is more often taken and administered by mouth or by injection. Common adverse effects include nausea and rash.

The medication and dose depend on whether your infection is complicated or uncomplicated. "Uncomplicated" means your urinary tract is normal, but you have a few symptoms, whereas "complicated" suggests you have an illness or problem with it.

A constriction of ureters, tubes that transport urine from your kidneys to your bladder, is the urethra, which transports urine from the bladder out of the body, narrows, or blockages like a kidney stone and enlarged prostate are all possibilities.

Your doctor may prescribe a more significant dose of antibiotics to treat complicated infections. But if your UTI continues to worsen and will reach the condition where it is severe, or the disease has spread to your kidneys, you may need to be treated in a hospital or doctor's office with high-dose antibiotics administered by IV.

Before prescribing you an antibiotic, your doctor's primary concern is to consider all the necessary factors. They carefully asked typical questions like this;

Are you pregnant?

Are you over 65 years old?

Are you allergic to any antibiotics?

Have you ever had any side effects from antibiotics in the past?

When we take antibiotics, we usually have a few questions. How long should antibiotics be taken? Antibiotics are generally prescribed for 2 to 3 days for a superficial infection.

These medications will be required for 7 to 10 days for some people because it usually depends on the severity of the tract infection. You may need to take antibiotics for 14 days or longer to ease the discomfort.

Your doctor will tell you if you need a follow-up urine test to see if the bacteria have gone away or not. If you still have an existing infection, you will be prescribed to continue taking antibiotics for a long time to avoid developing more severe problems.

How to feel better:

If your doctor has already prescribed you the best medicine to cure you, specifically antibiotics, this can give you relief. If you haven't visited a doctor yet, you can research online and buy over-the-counter medications like pain relievers. You must also take care of yourself by applying home remedies like taking enough vitamin c and practicing good sexual hygiene.

## Herbal Medicine for Treating Urinary Tract Infections.

Recurrent urinary tract infections are most common in women and can also be present in people of all ages. It can have a severe negative impact on the well-being of all. Although antibiotics are used to cure them, there are also many chances for recurring in some cases. It is very common to women.

In using preventive antibiotics, some specific issues and concerns are considered like; antibiotic resistance, side effects, and lack of long-term benefits from the treatments. So, some people believe in alternative medicine and treatments like Chinese Herbal Medicine.

Most Chinese medicines combine herbs, plants, vitamins, and root extracts. They always use natural ingredients and connect them to create effective drugs. The herbal remedy is most recommended for different illnesses such as UTI.

If you suspect that you have a bladder infection like UTI, you must consult a health care provider as soon as possible. What may start as a mild infection may lead to a serious problem if left untreated. The researcher found that 42% of benign and uncomplicated UTIs can be resolved without antibiotics or any drugs.

Here are some examples of Herbs and Natural Supplements that may help prevent or treat mild UTIs:

1) D-mannose is a naturally occurring sugar that may help treat urinary tract infections by preventing infectious bacteria from adhering to cells in the urinary system. Early study suggests it could treat and prevent UTIs, but additional research is needed.
2) Uva Ursi (Bearberry leaf) - Otherwise known as Arctostaphylos uva ursi or bearberry leaf - is an herbal remedy for UTIs that has been used in traditional medicine practices for centuries.
3) Garlic is a well-known herb that has been utilized in culinary and traditional medical techniques for centuries.
4) Cranberry products, such as juices and extracts, are among the most popular natural and alternative treatments for urinary tract infections.
5) Green Tea: This is made from the leaves of the Camellia sinensis plant. It has been employed in many traditional medicine systems for millennia due to its vast pharmacological potential.
6) Parsley Tea: Parsley has a slight diuretic effect, which is thought to help drain bacteria that cause UTIs out of the urinary tract.
7) Chamomile Tea: Chamomile tea is used in herbal therapy to treat various diseases, including urinary tract infections.
8) Teas produced from peppermint and other species of wild mint are occasionally used as a natural cure for UTIs.

## Flotrol Natural Bladder Support Supplements

If you are suffering from discomfort, pain, embarrassment due to your bladder, this is the answer to your problem. Flotrol is a 100% natural ingredient product that can help people with an Overactive Bladder. The team of Flotrol developed this fantastic product that is super affordable and easy to purchase.

The potent plant extracts in the form of easy-to-swallow capsules are within your reach. You don't need a prescription to buy this product. All you have to do is place an order online, and it will be delivered at the convenience of your doorstep.

It comes from an affordable package deal that is super friendly in your pocket. You will receive many packages as your purchase (2 bottles- 60 capsules).

By using this fantastic product, you will experience relief in days. Imagine your life free of worries about your bladder again. You can do activities without worrying about leakage, the sudden urge to urinate, and embarrassing incidents. You can travel again, go shopping, enjoy a friend's company over the weekend and, like me, Date without interruption again.

Flotrol ingredients are clinically proven, beneficial to your health and body. It helps you strengthen and rejuvenate your bladder. The combination of pumpkin seeds and soy is so unique that it can cure bladder problems. This product is a breakthrough that can help you with your overactive bladder.

If you suffer from overactive bladder syndrome and probably experiencing symptoms like the following:

- I need to go to the restroom urgently with little warning.
- I am not being able to hold or control your urine.
- Leakage before or after you have urinated.
- I have to pee at least 6 to 8 times per day.

This product is perfect for you. It will make your life easy, and you will have the liberty to do the things you are doing before you have this problem. Using it will allow you to trust your bladder again, and your social life will be back to its former glory.

You don't need to worry about having to find the nearest restroom or if you can get to it in time. Based on my personal experience after using the product, I don't need to worry if Mari and I are having a date.

I enjoy her company at the last minute when we are together. Flotrol is a lifesaver for me. It also helps me to recover my self-confidence of being manly again.

About the Product:

Flotrol Natural Bladder Support is made of Natural Herbal ingredients that are very friendly to your body. You don't need to worry about side effects, and it is easy to take it because of the soft gel capsule.

Here are the things you need to know about Flotrol:

- Contains Pumpkin seeds and soy extract - We all know we can trust ancient medicine. Pumpkin seeds were used traditionally by Native American Tribes during the 15th century to cure bladder problems. Scientifically it is approved to treat irritable bladder. With the combination of soy extract, it is very effective to regulate your bladder problems.
- Supports Bladder control naturally - Because of its natural ingredients, it will indeed work in your system. Taking the right amount in your daily dose will help control your irritated and overactive bladder right away. It is very safe to use and very reliable too.
- No prescription needed- Because of its natural ingredients, you can purchase it hassle-free because no prescription is required. All you need to do is order it, and it will be delivered to your doorstep without any delay.
- Easy to swallow capsules - Some people have a complex, time-consuming medicine, especially capsule form. The frontal is a supplement in a unique form; that is why anyone will easily swallow it.
- Specially formulated for mature adults - Men and women of older ages are most prone to bladder problems. This product is specially made for mature users. With its natural ingredients, it is very safe for them to use.
- It helps you avoid sleepless nights and embarrassing accidents - Having an overactive bladder is very discomforting. Undeniable trips to the restroom more than eight times per night as if it is endless. Most of the time, people who have bladder issues are often caught in embarrassing situations or incidents. Using this product, you can say goodbye to it all.
- Made in the USA - Everybody knows that it is proven and tested if made in the US... It is well studied, and it passes all the necessary qualities that are very safe to use. The US-

made is very reliable and with good standard.

Million all over the world are affected by bladder problems. Old age is one reason for loss of bladder control. To add up, unhealthy lifestyles and vices like smoking and drinking can also make it worst. It can affect the bladder muscles that can lead to urinary incontinence.

Flotrol is clinically proven to strengthen the weakened muscles that keep the urine flow under control. According to studies, people using the product felt better after 3 days of constant use. It is a lifesaver to those who suffer from bladder problems.

It is a dietary supplement made from herbal ingredients (pumpkin seeds and soy extract) to strengthen the bladder. The formula works to repair and maintain the walls of your bladder, enabling it to contract and usually relax and to urinate normally.

It helps improve your urinary tract, and using it will help your overactive Bladder function typically. It can be used by both men and women of a certain age, and it is very safe and very effective in treating involuntary leakage of your urine. The study found a marked improvement in urinary tract health and overall quality of life.

Here are some essential details about Flotrol:

How does it work?

Flotrol essentially works by strengthening your bladder muscles. It also helps to improve your urinary tract health. For men of old age, it is proven to help improve prostate health that will help avoid some risk in developing prostate problems.

Advantages:

1) The formula is clinically proven and very effective.
2) It has all the natural formulation with no side effects.
3) There are many good reviews and feedback from those who have tried the product.
4) It improves your overall tract health, and it is clinically proven to strengthen the walls of your bladder.

Dosage suggestions:

Take five tablets a day with meals for two weeks, then reduce to three pills a day for maintenance starting the third week.

Flotrol was created in 2002 by a company that is a proud member of the Natural Products Association. The company is committed to its mission of offering practical and safe health and wellness solutions. Also, the product was made initially in the United States of America. It's available for purchase on the brand's official website.

With Flotrol, you can now control your life and your bladder as well. Live your life as you desire. Travel, go out with friends, spend your time outdoors, watch a football game, enjoy weekends with loved ones at the beach, Date again, among other things. I am telling you, Flotrol is worth a try.

# Chapter 20:
# Who Is Most Prone to This Kind of Problem?

Bladder Infections and UTIs can affect men and women of all ages, including babies. However, women are more likely to be involved. If a certain bacteria enters our system, our bodies typically react. We develop indications and symptoms as our bodies ingest it and our antibodies react.

In most cases, infections are caused by Escherichia coli, which lives in the intestine. In the event when E. From the rectum to the vaginal canal, E. coli can enter the urethra and infect the bladder.

The age-related risk factors for UTI differ. Sexual intercourse and the use of spermicides are the most common risk factors before menopause. Sex increases the number of bacteria in the bladder; thus, many specialists recommend that women urinate after sex to wash them out.

Lactobacilli, which are good in the vaginal environment, maybe killed by spermicides—making it easier for E. coli to take up residence. Specific anatomical changes that occur during menopause assist in setting the setting for UTIs. The amount of Lactobacilli in the vaginal canal naturally decreases.

In addition, the bladder contracts less powerfully than it did previously, making it more difficult to empty. Genes play a role in both premenopausal and postmenopausal women. Having a mother or sibling who suffers from UTIs regularly is also a risk factor.

The most frequently asked question is, "Why are women more susceptible to and at risk for bladder infections?" Unfortunately, statistics show that more than half of women worldwide will have UTIs at some point in their lives.

This stealthy illness, which causes bothersome symptoms including painful abdominal urination and frequent urine, might return if any of the following two things occur:

- At first, conventional/home treatments for infection suppression appear to work, but they don't.
- A different strain of germs is exposed to the woman. Even still, none of this explains why women are more susceptible to urinary infections. Anyone or a combination of these variables could be to blame.

There are a few fundamental reasons why children develop UTIs.

1) Bacteria from a child's skin can enter the urinary tract and cause infections. It's important to consider how youngsters wipe after using the restroom.
2) A child's urinary tract is positioned to be more susceptible to contracting a UTI. Children pick up "poor habits" like holding their urine too long or racing out of the bathroom.
3) By modifying specific behaviors, you can help your child lower their risk of becoming infected.

Here are critical ideas that can help your child develop good restroom habits, which may help prevent infections later on:

- Use the potty more often. Young children hold their pee for extended periods because they do not like to take breaks from playing. Some children, who have experienced a UTI in the past, are afraid to pee because they think it will hurt again. When I ask my 4-year-old nephew if he needs to use the potty, the answer is almost always "NO." However, he can constantly pee when I take him to the bathroom. Sound familiar?
- Rather than asking, tell your youngster when it's time to go to the bathroom. Make it a need rather than a choice. We recommend that youngsters empty their bladders every two to three hours at the absolute least. When urine remains in the bladder for an extended period, bacteria can proliferate and infect.
- Time your child's potty sessions. Children need to stay on a timed schedule for using the bathroom to make sure they empty their bladders often. I recommend that parents program a "toilet watch" to buzz or vibrate at a certain period

during the day. Because they are inconspicuous, the vibrating ones are ideal for older school-aged youngsters. If you type "toilet watch" into your favorite search engine, you'll get a variety of results. Phone alarms can be configured to vibrate or do the same for older children and teens.

- Proper wiping. Wipe front to back. It's also critical that your youngster understands that toilet tissue used to wipe their bottom should not be utilized to wipe their urethral area (where pee comes out).

- Choices in clothing. Cotton underwear is preferred, especially in the summer, because they allow air to circulate beneath them. Also, tight clothes, such as narrow jeans, do not allow enough circulation, allowing bacteria to thrive and create an infection. If your child has trouble controlling themselves when they go to the bathroom, they should frequently change their underwear since dampness encourages bacteria to develop, leading to infection.

- There will be no bubble baths. All youngsters should avoid taking bubble baths with foamy soap since it might cause skin irritation on and around the genitalia. Showers or ordinary baths are acceptable options.

- Keep yourself hydrated. Urine should have a pale-yellow tone, almost transparent. The more your youngster drinks, the more frequently they need to use the restroom. When the bladder is washed out often, it is happy and healthiest. Dark urine burns more efficiently, making a child want to keep their urine inside.

- Children who keep their stools and have their urine should not be constipated. Bacteria are closer to the urethra when the chair is found in the lower region of the colon (where pee comes out). Once a day, we recommend that children have a bowel                                                  movement. Remove the bladder and empty it. After peeing, some children may not empty their bladder. They urinate just enough to get rid of the sensation because they're in a rush to get back to what we're doing or because they're so used to holding on to their urine that their body tightens the bladder muscles in the middle of peeing, causing them to stop too soon. Each time your youngster goes to the bathroom, tell them to "double pee." Double peeing is when someone tries to urinate twice after having already peed to promote bladder emptying.

Urinary tract infections are not fun, but fortunately for all of us, they can be preventable. I hope you find helpful tips, and I encourage you to share this with other parents.

# Reasons Why Women are More Prone to UTI than Men

### 1. Structure of the human body

When germs from the external genitals and the area around the anus enter the urinary tract and reach the bladder, women acquire UTI. E. E. coli bacteria are naturally present in certain places, placing women in greater danger.

Bacteria can easily access the urinary tract because the urethra, which transports urine out of the bladder, is short. The contamination of the perineum area (between the anus and external genitals) and the urethral area is the most likely cause of a urinary infection in women.

### 2. Sexual gratification

Intercourse decreases the germs and strains in the vaginal and urethral areas. Hence many women acquire a terrible case of Cystitis after being sexually active or having a new partner. Furthermore, microorganisms remain in the urinary tract when women do not urinate immediately after sex. It has the potential to cause them to multiply, resulting in infection.

Paying attention to excellent hygiene, especially when sexually active, can help women avoid UTI. Peeing after sex and cleaning the region regularly are two practices that can help lower the risk of infection.

### 3. Specific birth control methods are used.

Some forms of birth control, like spermicidal drugs and diaphragms, increase the risk of bladder infection in women. Nonoxynol-9, a hazardous ingredient found in most spermicides, has been linked to an increased risk of urinary infection. On the other hand, the diaphragm might damage the areas near the bladder, enabling germs easier to grip onto the inner linings.

## 4. Genetics

Yes, there is evidence that genetics may predispose women to urinary tract infections. A thorough analysis of one's family history can reveal a tight relationship between family members who have had recurring urine infections. It's because they have a higher density of certain carbohydrate receptors, which specific E. coli strains respond to. E. coli can adhere.

Unfortunately, there isn't much you can do if you feel your urinary infection is caused by genetics other than taking extra precautions. Also, get medical attention right away to minimize the severity of your UTI symptoms and effectively manage the disease.

## 5. Menopause

Bacteria in the urine, known as bacteriuria, affects 10 percent to 15 percent of women aged 65 to 70 and 20 percent to 50 percent of women aged 80 and beyond.

Assume the lady is in the premenopause stage and has a urinary infection such as cystitis or kidney issues. The disease is far more likely to return during the menopause and postmenopause periods if this is the case. Many factors could play here, including heredity, hormone changes, and age-related consequences from other conditions.

Hormonal changes caused by pregnancy can make women more sensitive to germs. It also causes anatomical alterations, albeit these are usually very transitory.

The enlarging and bulky uterus pulls on the bladder during pregnancy, making it more difficult for urine to exit the urinary canal. When urine remains in the bladder, it becomes a breeding ground for bacteria and puts the pregnant woman at increased risk of UTI.

Infections beginning in the urinary tract:

- A blockage anywhere in the urinary tract (for example, by stones).
- Neurologic illnesses cause abnormal bladder function, which hinders appropriate emptying.
- A urethral diverticulum, for instance, is a structural abnormality.
- When the valve-like mechanism between the ureter and the bladder leaks, urine and bacteria can travel backward from the bladder up the ureters and possibly into the kidneys (more common among children who have a UTI.)
- A doctor inserts a urinary catheter or any other tool.
- Sexual encounters
- Using a diaphragm in conjunction with spermicide.
- An inappropriate link (fistula) between the vaginal and bladder or the gut and the bladder is present.

# Chapter 21:
# Can Bladder Infection Be Prevented?

Others might say that having a bladder condition is hard to control and avoid. Also, because I have suffered from a bladder infection and almost ruined my Date, I never thought that a bladder infection could be prevented when appropriately treated.

How can you prevent UTIs?

- Don't hold your pee. Immediately go to the nearest bathroom as soon as you feel the urge to secrete urine.
- After urination, clean your private parts. You can rinse it with water or make sure to wipe it from front to back.
- Make a trip to the bathroom before and after sex.
- Enjoy baths? That's okay every once in a while, but take showers more often than you soak.
- Wear breathable underwear, preferably those made of cotton.
- Tight pants aren't in style for your pelvic health. Avoid wearing tight-fitting pants, and they can trap moisture.
- Drink plenty of water or keep yourself hydrated.

There are around a half-dozen oral antibiotics that can be used to treat UTIs. A doctor may prescribe one medicine and then switch to another once a urine culture reveals which bacterium is causing the infection. It may take time to adjust the medication, and recurrent infections occur.

Another infection develops quickly when a person feels better and decides to stop taking the Antibiotic despite the doctor's advice. Stopping antibiotics before your dose is finished is never a good idea.

Your doctor may prescribe an antibiotic to take before and after sexual activity if you're a younger lady who is sexually active. A vaginal estrogen cream for postmenopausal women may assist in preventing infections.

If the infections do not go away, your doctor may order tests to look for other health issues in the kidneys, bladder, or other parts of the urinary system.

Older folks are more aware of "retention issues," which become more prevalent as you become older. "I tell them to do a double-void — urinate and then urinate again." How about cranberry juice to help with UTIs? "There is contradicting research," she says. "It won't cure an illness, but use might help prevent one, so we don't discourage it."

If you've ever experienced a urinary tract infection, you understand how unpleasant and annoying the symptoms can be, especially when they strike at the worst possible time.

Urinary tract infections affect both men and women, as well as children.

Every year, the illness is said to cause more than 8.1 million visits to healthcare practitioners. While UTIs are simple to cure, they are also simple to avoid.

Let's take a deeper look at the best strategies to avoid a urinary tract infection and the accompanying painful and annoying symptoms.

Understanding where urinary tract infections come from is the most distinctive approach to thoroughly preventing them. The fundamental function of the urinary system, as you may know, is to produce and store urine. The Kidneys, Bladder, and Urethra are just a few elements that make up the urinary system.

Urine is produced in the kidneys, which are fist-sized organs in the back of the body that filter liquid waste from the blood and excrete it in urine.

It passes via the ureters and into the bladder, where it is kept until you feel the need to empty it. The urethra is used to discharge the urine—a tiny aperture above the vaginal opening or at the end of the penis.

Because the one-way flow prevents illnesses, normal urine contains no microorganisms. On the other hand, Bacteria can enter the urine through the urethra and migrate up into the bladder.

As a urinary tract infection progresses, it may spread to the kidneys, resulting in a more serious medical problem. A bladder infection is the most frequent kind of urinary tract infection.

If only we were equipped with so much knowledge about products that can help us prevent or relieve it from getting it worst, maybe we are all free from this kind of problem. Being well informed and having all the ideas about supplements that can help us resolve the overactive bladder is helpful for us. As the saying goes, "Prevention is better than cure. "

Flotrol is one product that can help you. It is a supplement that can promise to help you resolve the overactive bladder. With its natural ingredients that are derived from pumpkin seeds and soybean extract, it is very safe to use. It is also made especially for mature men and women.

# Chapter 22:
# The Proposal and the Wedding

## The Proposal:

It is the day, and it's now or never! I told myself that morning while facing the mirror. I am on the go for this. I feel good, look good, feel young, and am eager to do this now. The last attempt was very disappointing and devastating. It will be marked in the History, my life and will be told to the next generation of my family.

Jessie and Justin made the best arrangements. They are very hands-on on the upcoming event. They hired people to do amazing things, and it makes me happy because I know that Margaret will be proud of our children. They are both like Margaret junior, exact and keen on all the details.

When I called for help to them that I would propose to Mari again, they went ballistic and continued planning like I was not even around, lol. Jessie is like a boss, being the brain in our family, She is very uptight, and Justin and I just laugh because it seems like she is arguing with herself. All we can hear is, "Guys are we doing this or not.

It was jam-packed that night at the restaurant—too many customers. It was too loud due to the band that Jessie hired. I was so nervous that I was sweating like a horse, I don't know, but I felt like I had a heart attack. Even though the music and the people are too loud, I can hear my heartbeat. I can't feel my legs, and I am sweating all over. Waiting for Mari that night makes me sick to my stomach.

As Mari entered the restaurant, she looked so stunning in red. She is wearing the same dress she wore when I first saw her. "The Lady in Red "is the woman who sweeps me off my feet. She has no idea what will happen, and if she says yes, it will change our life together.

It is almost time, and the band is about to have their last song. Jessie and Justin, and the rest of the crew are ready. Then when the band was about to sing their last song, Jessie grabbed the mike and asked the couples if they wanted to dance along, and the best dance couple will win a prize. That was my cue!

I grab Mari and ask her to dance with me. She never hesitated, and we just went there and danced. As the band played the song, The Lady in red, I held the love of my life so tight that I didn't want to let her go. I can smell the fragrance I love and the woman who made me see beautiful things again. As I whispered to her ear, "I love You, "She just looked into my eyes and kissed me passionately.

Then Mari just suddenly notices, nobody is in the center but us; everyone is just looking at us, then she asks me, "Why are we the only two dancing"? Then I look at her, kneel, and ask her, "Mari Felicia Martinez, Will you spend the rest of your life with me? Will you marry me"? I can see the tears falling from her eyes while saying, "Yes, I will marry you!" And then She just kissed me to seal it.

## The Wedding:

After three months of preparation, the time has come. The weather is getting colder, and only two days before the wedding. All is well taken care of by my fabulous daughter. Ever since we planned the proposal, she just couldn't let it go and prepare for the wedding. Well, that's my girl, never argue with her.

It is just a simple church wedding as Mari is a catholic, and I have to respect her wishes to get married in a church. It was a solemn ceremony, and I was surprised that it was not that long. The next thing I knew was that the priest was already announcing us as man and wife.

I was so happy to have Mari as my wife. Yes, I have told her countless times how much I love her but being married is just a whole new level of happiness and fulfillment. It gave me goosebumps having to think how I get to call her my wife, and we get to spend the rest of our lives being each other's better halves.

Jessie and Justin's speech touched Mari and me during the reception. It even made me tear up a little because they really did accept Mari and never tried to look at her as a stranger but already a member of the family.

After the speeches, Mari and I got to have our first dance together, and can I just say that the medicines we are taking are effective because not once were we disturbed by an uncomfortable feeling to go to the bathroom during the duration of the party.

It was a lot to take in because looking back, and I couldn't believe that we were able to survive all of it together. Yes, I have been through a lot especially losing someone I love with all my heart, but Mari gave me a chance to feel like I can love again. She allowed me to feel like I could be okay again. She took the broken pieces of what was left of my heart, and she gladly glued them back together.

Then, just when I thought we would be happy, an illness similar to my condition struck the woman I fell in love with now. I almost wanted to scream and ask why I am experiencing all of these trials. But I was glad that I didn't give up.

As I held the hand of my beloved wife, I realized how lucky I was to have this person beside me. The one who stayed with me through it all. The pain, the hardships, the fear, and all those worries. Someone I know loves me as much as I love her and accepts me for who I am.

I look at Mari's eyes, and I can't help but feel emotional because this incredible woman right here agreed to spend the rest of her life with me. She vowed to love me and stay faithful to me for as long as we both shall live. She said "I do" to the part where the priest asked her if she would stay with me through sickness and health.

The way she smiled at my children melts my heart because you could see how her eyes glisten as if she were looking at her two most favorite people in the whole world. The way she cares for all of us reminds me how not all people get to have this kind of life. Not all get to enjoy the perks of having a peaceful life and being surrounded by the people who cherish and love you.

So, as we danced the night away, I was daydreaming of how our lives would look like, and I can say that whatever the future might bring us, I know I will be okay because I have Mari, Jessie, Justin, and the rest of the family beside me.

I leaned and whispered in her ear, "here's to the start of our kind of forever; I will love you, no matter what." She smiled the sweetest smile and kissed me. "Here's to us and our kind of perfect; I love you, too!" she replied.

Chills came down my spine because I couldn't believe what I heard. I pulled Mari closer and hugged her. It is my wife, and I will never let her go. It's her and me against the world for the rest of our life here on Earth.

The party ended pretty late, and we were exhausted from all the dancing and bonding with the family, but as we walked down the hallway going to our room, we smiled because we realized how we got through the night without any disturbances from our bladders. We both screamed, "Thank you, FLOTROL!"

I'm so glad that my wife will always be that one person who can understand me and my condition and won't ever get tired of taking care of me while she takes care of herself.

How did I get so lucky? As we prepared to sleep, I knew right then and there that Mari and I would have a great married life together. She just gets me without me having to explain what I need or what I want. She looks at me, and she instantly knows what I am feeling.

# Chapter 23:
# Conclusion

Having trouble with frequent urination can be annoying. It seems that some people find it very discomforting like me. I never thought that it could also be life-threatening if not medically treated.

It can cause more damage to your kidney and, of course, to your health. If a person is very busy and doesn't have time to take care of himself, more health problems can come their way. Complications make their way to make it more deadly.

Having this bladder condition was not easy for my family and me. Especially after my wife died and my new love suffered from a bladder problem, I was worried because these conditions are commonly heard but not taken seriously. It is happening to most of us at a certain age.

Not just to anyone I know, but to me personally. That is why I became more focused on my health and the health of my loved ones. I make sure that they take the necessary precautions, vitamins, and exercise as much as possible.

I talked to my children and grandchildren regularly to remind them that they should be more watchful with what they are eating and their way of living because I didn't want them to go through what I went through.

I keep telling them to avoid vices especially smoking, drinking, sleeping late, ignoring any signs and symptoms. I used to say, "Look what happened to Mari and me; we took ourselves for granted. " It is crucial to take care of yourself and make sure that you all watch what you are doing with it.

As other people say, "prevention is better than cure." So, I just want them to be as careful as possible because having a life free of illnesses and health conditions is what they should aim for themselves and their children. Life is precious, and we owe our life. We must be watchful and very keen on what we are feeling.

Having experienced that terrible bladder problem, Mari and I being husband and wife, always remind each other to be watchful and spread the excellent results that Flotrol brought us.

We never forget to take time to pause, exercise, eat healthily, keep hydrated, and take our daily supplements to take care of our bladder and our health as well.

It's been years that Mari and I haven't been bothered by our bladder problem. No more sleepless nights, pain, discomfort, and most of all, embarrassing moments. It is fantastic because we both get to do whatever we want, like traveling together with or without our family.

We are both enjoying a worry-free bladder life. The restaurant is doing well and going strong. Children and Grandchildren are happy and healthy with their lives. Mari and I grew old together and were contented and comfortable, and I couldn't ask for more.

I thank all who are behind Flotrol. You made my life more meaningful and beautiful with my wife, Mari. This fantastic product took away all my worries and sufferings. I am confident that it is very safe and effective to use natural ingredients.

Thank you, FLOTROL! I cannot imagine my life without you. Thank you for taking care of my wife and me. You gave me the best second chance with love and for bringing me back to my feet again.

It brought me back my confidence and my everyday life. My friendly advice to those experiencing and suffering from bladder problems: don't let your bladder control your life; never be afraid to ask for a second opinion or try supplements like Flotrol. If it works for Mari and me and the rest of us, I am sure it will work for you too.

Use the power of modern technology. Use your fingers and phone to search online, become aware of your body's condition, and find out what is best for you. Feel free and use the magic of the internet to search for Flotrol Natural Bladder Support Supplements; click their website, and I am sure you will learn more and be a happy customer. Money-back guaranteed.

Knowledge is power! The more aware you are, the more you learn. It is never too late for anything. Live your life to the fullest and enjoy without worry. Remember, we only have one life to live, so live it and don't just stop there; live it like there is no tomorrow!

But of course, you can try it for yourself too. In order to see if it works for you as much as it worked for me.

Here is the link https://bit.ly/flow399 and code for you to scan and get your own Flotrol at an affordable price:

SCAN ME